RECOVER FROM A STROKE

Also by Deborah Bleecker

Acupuncture Points Handbook
Virus Remedies Guidebook
Acupressure Made Simple
Tung Acupuncture Points
Acupuncture for Migraines
Shingles Relief
Natural Back Pain Solutions
Insomnia Relief

RECOVER FROM A STROKE

How Acupuncture, Acupressure, Natural Therapies, and Supplements Can Help You Recover

Deborah Bleecker, LAc, MSOM

Disclaimer

This book contains the opinions and ideas of the author. It is intended to provide helpful and informative material on the subjects addressed. It is sold with the understanding that the author and publisher are not engaged in rendering medical, health, psychological or any other type of advice or services in the book. If the reader needs personal, medical, health, or other assistance or advice, a competent professional should be consulted.

The author and publisher disclaim any responsibility for any liability, loss or risk, either personal or otherwise that occurs as a consequence, directly or indirectly, of the use and application of the contents of this book.

Draycott Publishing, LLC
0706 version

Tradepaper ISBN: 978-960096-82-1

Contents

Introduction

You are probably reading this book because you, or a loved one, has suffered a stroke, and you want to know what happened, and what you can do to help.

I have been there. In 1997 my dad had a stroke. I was in acupuncture school at the time, in another state, and only had a few days off from school to help him. I did not know what a stroke was, or what to do. I was able to help him recover quickly using basic principles of acupuncture and Chinese medicine, which are included in this book. There is nothing worse than watching your dad limp around the house, not knowing if he would ever walk normally again.

My mom had a stroke in 2021. I was allowed to treat her with acupuncture and other therapies while she was in the hospital. After two acupuncture treatments she was able to lift her affected arm again. She was also walking almost as well as before the stroke within a few days.

Acupuncture and acupressure can help the body recover after a stroke. It is always better to get treatment as soon as you can after a stroke, but your body continues to heal forever. The longer it has been since the stroke, the longer it will take to get better. Treating sooner also helps to prevent new problems from occurring.

You can treat yourself while lying in bed. Simply activate the acupuncture points, and your body does the rest. You do not have to believe that it works.

Your Life is Not Over

If you had a stroke, you might feel your life is over. You don't know how you will recover. You think you might not recover. This is a normal feeling after you suffer a serious health problem. We always think there is no way our body will heal. The human body is a self-healing organism. You are healing every day. Most people believe they will not recover from many health problems that are easy to treat with Chinese medicine. Licensed Acupuncturists treat "incurable" illnesses every day.

It is Never Too Late

The goal of this book is to help you recover much faster than you would otherwise. It does not matter when you had your stroke. You are always healing. There is no time limit on healing.

I treated a man who had his stroke as a teenager, 18 years prior to seeing me. I told him that I did not know if I could help him, but I was willing to try. Most doctors told him that he was past the time period he could improve. He walked with a limp, and he wanted to walk better. Acupuncture helped him to improve his walking after a series of treatments. It is never too late.

I know what it is like to be written off, and told that it is not possible to recover from health issues. I had that experience before I started acupuncture school. Because of that, I would never tell someone there was no chance of improvement.

The Purpose of This Book

Since most people do not have access to acupuncture at this time, I have included all the points you need to know to treat yourself, or have someone else treat you with acupressure, and other modalities. There are 146 images in this book.

You cannot depend on other people. You need to help yourself. But you need to know what areas to treat, to address all your health issues.

If you don't want to read the text, you don't have to. You can just look at the images and press firmly, or use other acupressure techniques listed in this book, like a mini massager.

I believe it will not take as long as you think to get results. You will not be treating these points a long time. You should feel a difference within a few days.

Real Points That Work

Most acupressure books are written by people who are not even acupuncturists. I have even seen a bestselling acupressure book where the information was completely made up by the author, and you would get no benefit from using that. Please be careful who you get advice from. Always insist on knowing points numbers, or names. I have a degree in Chinese medicine, and have been using acupuncture for 30 years now. These points work.

You Can Help Yourself While Lying in a Hospital Bed

Easy to Understand Stroke Explanation

When my dad had his stroke, in 1997, I had to figure out how to explain to myself what happened, so I would know what to do. There was no book on how to treat strokes with acupuncture. This book is the only book I am aware of that includes how to treat strokes from head to toe, with acupuncture, acupressure, and supplements.

Stimulating acupuncture points sends signals to the brain, to wake it up. In a way, your brain does not recognize the part of your body that has been affected by the stroke.

Stimulating points in your hand, sends signals to your brain to wake up, and start controlling the hand again.

For example, if you have a problem with incontinence, points that regulate the bladder can be treated. That wakes the bladder up, and the brain now sends effective signals to the bladder.

If you have a problem lifting your arm, you treat the muscles on your shoulder that lift your arm. This sends a signal to your brain, to make it recognize those muscles again.

Press each point for three to five minutes. If the sensation is too intense, stop treating the point. A mini massager is the best choice, but you can use your fingers, and ear seeds. Everything you need to know is explained in the how to make acupressure work chapter.

If you cannot speak or swallow, there are specific acupuncture points that send signals to the brain to restore healthy function. It is very simple, and very beautiful.

If you think treating strokes with these techniques cannot work, think about what happens to your hand when you touch a hot stove. Your hand sends a signal to the brain, and the brain quickly tells you to move your hand. The nerves in your hand are connected to your brain. It is a feedback loop.

The brain tells the body to move the hand. The hand sends signals to the brain at all times. It is connected. This connection is called reflex action.

Most points are self-explanatory. You do not have to read the text. You can just start using the points as shown in the image, and the points are easy to find.

Acupuncture is Unbelievable

You are probably thinking that there is no way acupuncture, or acupressure could help you recover faster from a stroke. Most of what acupuncture and Chinese herbs do is unbelievable.

Even I am shocked on a regular basis, and I have been using acupuncture points for 30 years now. Acupressure works, when done on the right points, and when the points are activated fully. I get plenty of feedback from readers of my acupressure book, *Acupressure Made Simple,* that people are able to help themselves with their health issues.

If you would like to see acupuncture being used to help a stroke patient, you can look online to find a documentary called *9,000 Needles*. At the time of this writing, it is available for streaming on Amazon. The release year was 2009.

CHAPTER 1

PHYSICAL EFFECTS OF A STROKE

The standard acronym, to be able to recognize a stroke is BEFAST.
B is for balance. You might fall.
E is for eyes, any change in vision.
F is for face, you might see a droop, or an uneven smile.
A is for arms, you might have arm numbness, or weakness. Ask the patient to lift the arms.
S is for Speech difficulty, which can include slurred speech, or difficulty understanding speech.
T is for time. If any of these symptoms is present, even if they come and go, call 911 to get immediate help.

Other possible symptoms of a stroke include:

- Sudden numbness
- Sudden confusion
- Sudden trouble seeing
- Sudden trouble walking
- Sudden severe headache

Some doctors expect that recovery from stroke occurs only in the first three to six months. In fact, I have heard that some doctors tell their patients that if they have not fully recovered within six months, that they will not improve from that point. That is not true. If you continue to work towards your recovery, you will continue to improve. The theory that stroke recovery is limited to six months is an old theory. It is never too late.

If someone tells you that you will not continue to improve, you should ignore that person. I had a nerve injury in 1994, and went from doctor to doctor to find help, and they all told me that my nerve problem was incurable. I did not accept that idea. I started studying natural medicine, and started acupuncture school in 1996. I resolved my health problems using Chinese medicine, and you can too.

The following statistics are depressing. It is hard to read how many people have strokes, and the long-lasting damage they suffer. I believe that everyone who has a stroke should start acupuncture treatment as soon as possible. The sooner you start treatment, the faster you recover. Although you can always benefit from acupuncture. These issues are treated by using the information in this book.

There are about 7 million stroke survivors in the United States, as of 2023, and about 133 million worldwide.

Common issues include:

- Mental issues
- Depression
- Personality changes
- Vision
- Hearing
- Speaking
- Swallowing

Seizures occur in about 6 to 15 % of stroke patients during the first week after a stroke. Deep vein thrombosis occurs in about 14% of patients during the first two weeks. Stroke related pain occurs in 21% of stroke survivors.

Vision problems occur in 93% of stroke survivors. People often do not know they have a vision problem until they get an eye exam.

Difficulty swallowing occurs in about 45% of stroke patients. When first admitted to the hospital, they will not allow you to drink or eat until you have been assessed for this problem. If you have difficulty swallowing, the food or drink can go down your windpipe, and you could suffocate.

About 25 to 43% of survivors will have spasticity in the first year after their stroke. It's more common in younger stroke survivors. It's also more common when the stroke is caused by a bleed (hemorrhagic stroke). The timing of spasticity occurring after a stroke can vary. From www.Stroke.org.

Blood Thinners

Blood thinning drugs might not be started immediately after a stroke. Typically, these drugs are started 7-14 days post stroke. Doctors have to be careful before deciding to start blood thinners. There is a risk of a hemorrhagic stroke. Factors they consider before starting this are size of the stroke infarcted area, location, atrial fibrillation, embolism, high blood sugar, low platelet count, and poor collateral circulation.

Complications after a Stroke

The incidence of complications after a stroke include:

Urinary Tract infection	24%
Pneumonia	22%
Pressure sores	21%
Depression	16%
Anxiety	14%
Another stroke	9%
Epileptic seizure	3%
Deep vein thrombosis	2%
Pulmonary embolism	1%

Source: Langhorne P, Stott DJ, Robertson L, MacDonald J, Jones L, McAlpine C, Dick F, Taylor GS, Murray G. Medical complications after stroke: a multicenter study. Stroke. 2000 Jun;31(6):1223-9. doi: 10.1161/01.str.31.6.1223. PMID: 10835436.

Physical effects of stroke can include:

- Aphasia, difficulty speaking and understanding speech
- Balance problems
- Bladder and bowel problems
- Changes in sensation
- Changes to taste and smell
- Fatigue (extreme tiredness)
- Foot drop (difficulty lifting your foot and toes)
- Headaches
- Muscle weakness.
- Pain
- Seizures and epilepsy
- Spasticity and contractures (muscle stiffness)
- Swallowing problems

- Vision problems

Foot Drop

Foot drop can cause your toes to catch on the ground when you step forward. You may lift your foot higher than usual when walking, or swing the leg outwards. This is due to weakness in muscle groups in the foot and ankle that lift your foot. It can lead to difficulty walking, and a higher chance of falling. They say that each stroke is unique, no two strokes are alike

Fatigue

After a stroke, many people have fatigue that does not get better with rest. You may find that you lose your grip and objects slip out of your hand. You might tire more easily than before your stroke.

Pain

You might suffer from pain, spasticity, and muscle tightness. Shoulder pain, which can be caused by muscle stiffness, or because weak muscles lead to a partial dislocation. Some patients have sensations such as tingling, cold, or burning, which might be a result of damage to the nervous system. You might have headaches.

Spasticity

In spasticity, the muscles are tight. This affects about one third of patients. Spasticity can develop within a week of a stroke, or later. I believe that getting acupuncture, or acupressure can make spasticity less likely. My explanation of it is that it is caused by your brain trying to send signals to an area that cannot process them.

Contractures

Spasticity can sometimes cause a permanent shortening of the muscles, called contracture. Muscles can become shorter, or longer. This can also cause the joints to become fixed in position. This can mean that the joint cannot be fully bent or straightened, and the muscles cannot be stretched to their full length.

The following section is taken directly from the website. These are the exact words they used. I strongly suggest you visit their website at www.stroke.org.uk for further information. This was one of the best resources I found for the physical effects of a stroke.

- **Feeling less sensitive to touch.** This is called hypoesthesia. Your limbs may feel numb and this can cause difficulties. For example, if you are unaware of pressure on your skin, such as tight clothing or shoes, they might rub and damage your skin without you noticing.
- **Feeling less sensitive to temperature.** If you experience this you could be at risk of burning yourself or becoming too cold, so you may need to take extra measures to look after yourself. For example, you might need to carefully test water temperatures with your good hand if having a shower or when washing up.

- **Feeling more sensitive to stimuli.** This is called hyperesthesia and can affect a range of your senses such as your taste, hearing or touch. After a stroke, some people find watching television or being in crowded places difficult as they seem too loud.
- **Feeling unaware of the position and movement of your limbs.** Your body has a system that makes it aware of its position and movement. Some people have problems with this after a stroke. If this is the case for you, you may have difficulty moving around, and you might find that you need to look at your limbs to know where they are. Some people feel as if their limbs (or part of them) feel like they do not belong to them, or like they have altered size or shape.
- **Having unusual sensations on your skin or in your limbs.** This is sometimes called dysesthesia or paresthesia. Common sensations are pins and needles or tingling in your affected limbs. Sometimes these sensations can be unpleasant, such as burning, pressure or feeling like something is running over your skin.

CHAPTER 2

STROKE STATISTICS

The purpose of this chapter is to give you a little information on what medical care costs to treat stroke patients. This information is available online, but please consult a professional to determine what your personal financial exposure is.

You will have a better understanding of what is going to happen to you in the hospital. For example, my mom was transferred to rehab after a few days in the hospital, and she was allowed to stay for 20 days. She had 20 days, because that is what Medicare usually covers.

I believe that if every rehab facility had a Licensed Acupuncturist on staff, patients would recover much more quickly, and be able to return to their homes, and have a better outcome.

Why Stroke Rehabilitation Centers Need Licensed Acupuncturists

Your Licensed Acupuncturist could help you locate the acupressure points and make sure every issue is addressed, in cooperation with your physical therapists and other staff. Your acupuncturist could also treat you with acupuncture to speed your recovery. In between acupuncture treatments, you could help yourself with acupressure.

The estimated annual costs to treat strokes is about $103 Billion dollars in the U.S. Indirect costs such as lost wages, and the loss of the ability to work is estimated at $17 to $38 billion per year.

Worldwide, there are almost 12 million new strokes each year. Globally, one in four people above age 25 years will have a stroke in their lifetime. Each year, about 15% of all strokes occur in people 15–49 years of age. Each year, about 53% of all strokes occur in people below 70 years of age.

There are 800,000 strokes in the United States each year. 65% of those living with stroke also suffer a disability that impedes their ability to carry out daily living.

After a stroke, you will need to be in a rehab facility, because they know how to help you walk safely, and can provide what you need. You will have 20 days to get well as fast as possible, before you are sent home, unless you can pay for extra days on your own.

Medicare Coverage, and What Patients Pay

The annual cost to Medicare for stroke care averages about **$47,000 per beneficiary** in the first year following an ischemic (blood clot) stroke. The specific costs to both Medicare and the patient vary based on the severity of the stroke, and the types of care required.

Medicare pays about $20,000 for the initial hospitalization of stroke patients. Rehabilitation care averages $17,000 per year.

For a nondisabling stroke, Medicare pays about $10,192 per patient, and the patient pays around $2,038.

For a moderately disabling stroke Medicare pays about $50,798, and the patient pays about $18,000.

For a severely disabling stroke Medicare pays about $83,000, and the patients pays about $48,000.

Part A Hospitalization costs for days 1-60 there is no copay. For days 61-90, the patient pays $419 per day.

A skilled nursing facility is covered 100% for the first 20 days, for days 21 to 100 there is a daily coinsurance of $209.50. There are also therapy limit caps.

These figures are approximate, and the year is 2026.

Cost to Provide Acupuncture in Rehabilitation Facilities

Let's see how acupuncture could help not only restore people's health faster after a stroke, but also save the medical system money in the long run.

Private acupuncture treatments cost about $100. After patients leave the rehabilitation facility, it can be hard for them to get transportation to their appointments.

To restore function in the limbs, expect at least 12 treatments if given soon after the stroke. If you have other issues, allocate at least three treatments per issue.

If a rehabilitation center, or hospital hired a Licensed Acupuncturist and paid him or her about $10,000 per month in salary, that would amount to about $15.62 per patient treatment. Since each stroke patient has different issues, it is hard to estimate the total number of treatments needed. But let's say you treated:

- Shoulder, to be able to lift the arm, 3 treatments
- Elbow, forearm, and hand, to be able to write again, 3 treatments
- Hip, leg, 3 treatments, walking

- Knees, lower leg, foot, 3 treatments, walking

If the treatments are given soon after the stroke, and combined with physical therapy, that would be 12 treatments, which totals $187.44 per patient, for the first week of acupuncture care. Keep in mind that a Licensed Acupuncturist could treat three to four patients per hour. It is a very cost-effective type of therapy.

If the patient has swallowing problems, constipation, incontinence, or other health issues, that can be addressed also. Treating the patient in the rehabilitation facility, soon after the stroke, will help the person recover much faster, while he or she has access to medical help.

So, for less than $200, stroke patients can benefit from accelerated recovery, and a whole week of daily acupuncture treatments. All we need to do to make this happen, is for patients to ask their rehab facility to hire Licensed Acupuncturists to work for them.

The problem right now is that most people have no idea how amazing acupuncture is, so the facility owners and managers don't think of having Licensed Acupuncturists on staff.

Acupuncturists cannot walk into a facility and treat patients in hospitals or rehab centers. The facility has to give them written permission to do so. The facility is responsible for the health and safety of its patients, and outside practitioners are not allowed to treat without approval. They have to do a background check to verify licensing, which is called credentialing.

In addition, Medicare does not cover acupuncture right now, so facilities would not be compensated for acupuncture. It is not only life altering for stroke patients, but it also saves money in the short and long term by helping the patients recover more quickly and require fewer other services at a later time.

Chapter 3

HOW TO MAKE ACUPRESSURE WORK

Acupressure is simply pressing on, or massaging acupuncture points to activate them, instead of inserting needles. When acupuncture is done, the needles are inserted, and they remain in place for about 30 minutes. During that time, the body is processing the point.

Just pressing the point for a few seconds is rarely enough to activate it. There is an expression in Chinese medicine called "getting the Qi". That means that you have stimulated the point enough that it has now been activated, and it is working.

Once the point is activated, you will usually notice a sensation in the point. Sometimes you do not feel anything. And some points feel stronger than others, because of their nature, and location. But the point needs to be stimulated enough to be activated. Treat the affected side. The points are on both sides of the body, except the Ren and Du meridians. When treating internal disorders, treat the healthy side.

Fake Acupressure

As an acupuncturist, I cringe when I see non-acupuncturists telling people to press on the point for five seconds. There are also a lot of acupressure books written by people who are not acupuncturists. They just make things up. The problem with this is that you will get no benefit, and you will blame acupressure in general, not the book written by someone who just makes things up. I wrote my own acupressure book, because I wanted people to have a book that told the truth. That book is called *Acupressure Made Simple*.

The point images are labeled with the point numbers, using an abbreviation of the meridian. The reason for this is that you can refer to the text and confirm the name of the point and what it is doing. If you do research on acupuncture, or acupressure, make sure the person tells you the point number. This should include the meridian, and number, or point name. There is a lot of made-up information online and in books. You should be able to cross reference.

To get the most accurate information, I cross-referenced every acupuncture point book I had against online references to write my book, *Acupuncture Points Handbook*. The location and functions of each point were taken from my book. For this book, I explain each point in reference to the reason the point is being used. So if one point has 30 functions, I will not list all the functions, only the functions that apply to stroke recovery. Some points have several pages of functions and indications, which are not always relevant to help you recover from a stroke.

The Images Are Easy to Understand

The images are labeled with the area, or issue, being treated. If space allowed, I included the point names. You don't have to know the point names or functions. Just look at the images and get started with your acupressure. Points on the face are the fastest to work, it sometimes only takes a minute for them to be activated.

If you treat a point, and feel uncomfortable, stop treating it. Especially with a massager, you might need little time to get results. You do not need to continue treating once the point is activated.

Getting the Qi

Once a point has been activated, you might be able to feel it. Although the sensation with acupressure is much less than when using acupuncture needles, you might still feel something.

If you are treating an area that has been affected by a stroke, you might not feel this sensation at all, until the points wake up. The sensations include numbness, tingling, itching, swelling, and a sensation that something is going on in the area. This is your goal. You want to feel something.

I have noticed that acupressure on the face causes a very strong itching sensation, when using a mini massager. Points on the leg are more likely to cause a swelling or achy feeling. You might still feel nothing at all, because you might not know what sensation you are looking for. So don't despair. Just spend the time you need to stimulate the point for 3-5 minutes, then move on to the next point.

You might treat the points three times, and feel nothing, then on the fourth treatment you feel it, and get results. The points have to be woken up.

Be Patient about How Much Time It Takes to Heal

You might not feel anything different for a while after the treatment. Some effects are fast, sometimes you feel something in a few hours, sometimes you notice something the next day. I treated my mom's arm with acupuncture after her stroke, and she was able to raise her arm again after the second treatment. Everyone will be different.

I would personally treat an issue twice a day for five days. Then switch to once a day. I would expect some improvement in the first five days.

If new problems occur, just treat the points in the affected area again. Healing is a process. If you get acupuncture from a Licensed Acupuncturist, he or she will have a preferred protocol and will be able to adjust your treatment according to how you respond. There is no protocol set in stone, it is important to be flexible and adapt to your specific situation.

To stimulate acupuncture points you can:

- Press or massage with your fingertips
- Use a mini massager
- Use ear seeds, which are Vaccaria seeds on surgical tape. If you press firmly on an acupuncture point with an ear seed in it, it almost feels like inserting a needle
- Use the tip of a Sonicare toothbrush to activate the points

This mini massager is easy to find online. It comes with different caps. You can use the smooth cap to treat your face. If the stimulation is strong enough, you can use that cap for other areas. To treat locations other than the face, I prefer the cap with the most prongs for acupressure.

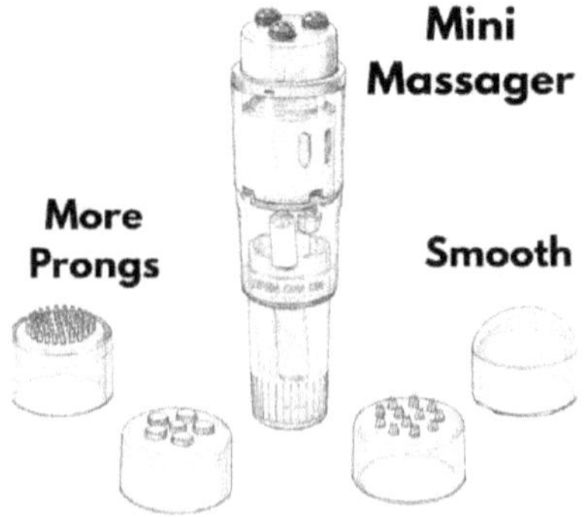

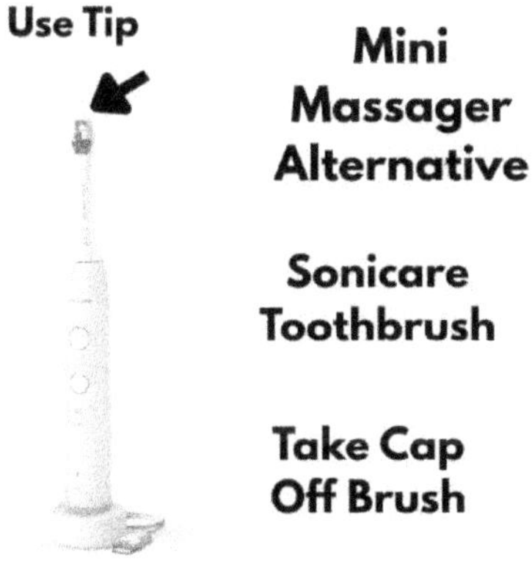

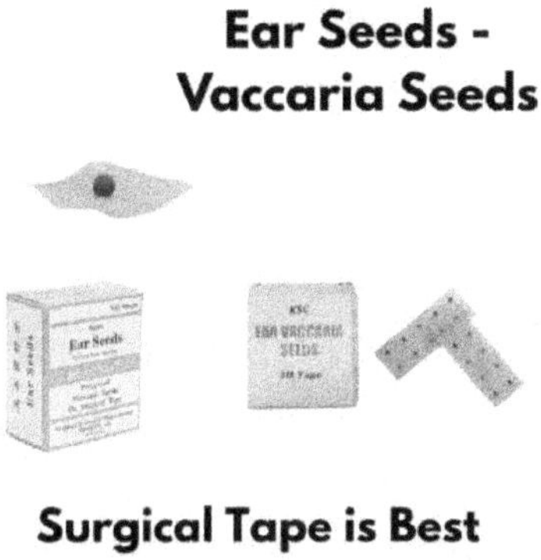

The prongs are smaller and seem to get a stronger effect. Using this cap on the face might increase the chance of breaking tiny blood vessels. It is not necessary to use a lot of stimulation on the face. I used the smooth tip for my face and it was very strong. It caused a lot of tingling. Once you get that sensation, you can stop treating that point. There is no need to continue stimulating the point.

The mini massager is about $10. Be sure to not buy a percussive massager. That could easily hurt you. You don't need strong stimulation.

Sonicare Toothbrush Can Be Used As a Massager

If you are not able to get a mini massager, I have found a great alternative, which you might already have. I tested my electric toothbrush tip with the cap off for acupressure and it was very effective. The Sonicare toothbrush vibrates and works great.

You might look silly using it, but who cares? You might already have this with you, and it is a good start to your healing. Take the cap off the brush, turn the toothbrush on, and use the tip of the brush to start your acupressure.

Acupuncture points are an area, not a pin point size. Don't worry about missing the point. When you do acupressure, you affect a larger area.

Oral Motor Stimulation Kit

In doing research to find effective ways to do acupressure, I ran across a device that is apparently used to help kids develop healthy mouth function. It is called an oral motor stimulation kit. It is less then half the size of a Sonicare toothbrush. It comes with multiple tips. You can use this device to get in smaller areas, such as between bones.

If you unscrew the attachment, the massager is stronger. You can use the edge of the tip for a very good point activation. I like it because it is lightweight, and the tip is a smaller diameter than most mini massagers, so you can get it into tighter areas, and the strength of the vibration is good. This massager is very strong, so be careful when using it on the face. Limit your time to a minute or two to avoid irritating nerves.

See a Licensed Acupuncturist, LAc

See an LAc. If you are able to get acupuncture by a Licensed Acupuncturist, I would do that as soon as possible. The person who treats you needs to have a degree in Chinese medicine, which is a three-year minimum master level program.

Licensed Acupuncturists spend an entire year learning where the points are located, how they work, how to combine them with other points, and how to be flexible on our point selection. We also learn needle insertion angle, and depth for each point.

I believe that Rehabilitation centers should have a Licensed Acupuncturist on staff. This will give patients a much faster and more complete recovery. Most people do not know how amazing acupuncture is at helping people recover faster, and more completely after a stroke.

I hope that you will spread the word to medical professionals on how it works.

Medicare Should Cover Acupuncture for Stroke Patients

I also believe Medicare and other insurance plans should cover acupuncture for stroke patients. Patients would recover more quickly if acupuncture could be combined with the physical therapy patients usually get. A Licensed Acupuncturist would be able to treat about four patients per hour.

Dry Needling is Not Acupuncture

Dry needling is not acupuncture. Dry needling is performed by people who do not have a degree in Chinese medicine. In many states, there is no training required, or a weekend class is all that is required. This is a horrible disservice to patients who do not know the difference, and do not recover, because the person was not trained properly.

I do not understand why any state would allow someone to insert acupuncture needles without a degree in Chinese medicine. It is dangerous, and it is often ineffective, and can cause damage to the tissue, which can easily cause additional trauma to overcome.

If you don't go to a dentist to get your colon checked, you should only see a Licensed Acupuncturist to get acupuncture.

In dry needling, they insert the needle, and fish around in the muscle for tight spots. This causes a lot of trauma to the muscle, which means you now have additional tissue damage to heal.

Some states only require a weekend class, which can be taken online, to do dry needling. Some people say they are "certified" in acupuncture or dry needling. That has no meaning in a legal sense. The companies that teach Dry Needling give their students a certificate of completion of the course. The course might be a weekend course, or two weekends.

Getting a state license requires a Master Degree in Chinese Medicine, which is currently a four-year program.

The term Dry Needling was coined by a Medical Doctor who injected trigger points in muscles to treat pain. She injected drugs with hypodermic needles, and when she did not use drugs, she called it a dry needling.

How Acupuncture Works

When acupuncture points are activated, a signal is sent to the brain via the acupuncture meridian. Each point has specific functions. If you have a fever, Large Intestine 11, by the elbow can be used to reduce it. If you have digestive issues, there are dozens of points to choose from, but Stomach 36 is always a good choice.

To treat pain, a Licensed Acupuncturist will determine which meridian is affected. Pain is caused by stagnation, which is a blockage of circulation.

Using the points, we can regulate the entire body, and relieve pain by restoring blood flow, as well as relaxing muscles and treating scar tissue that blocks healthy blood flow.

Acupuncture and Chinese herbs can treat you from head to toe. Acupressure can be amazing, and in some cases, I prefer using acupressure over using needles on myself. In some cases, I have found acupressure works faster than acupuncture.

Reflex System

The image below, showing the cactus, represents how when the end of the finger is stimulated, it sends a signal to the brain, and spine. This is how acupressure and acupuncture help you recover from a stroke. When the acupuncture points on the hand are stimulated, signals are sent to the brain, which then recognizes the hand again.

One way to understand it is that the hand is asleep, and the brain no longer recognizes it. The shoulder muscles are asleep, and the brain cannot send signals strong enough to lift your arm. The muscles that lift the arm are located in the shoulder. The muscles that move the fingers are located in the forearm and fingers. When you treat all affected areas, you can restore full function.

Physical therapy is very important to recover after a stroke. But acupuncture speeds up the time it takes for the brain to remember the affected side of the body. The points are located from the top of your head to the tips of your toes. Activating these points will help your brain to restore function much faster than anything else.

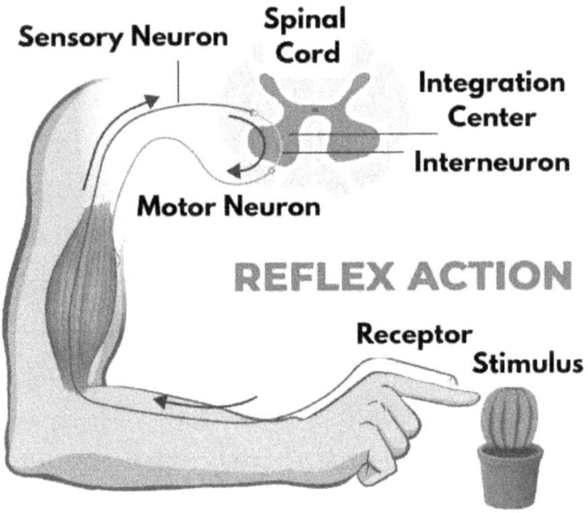

Stimulating a point on your hand, large intestine 4, opens the entire meridian, which ends by your nose.

You can treat points on your foot, on your stomach meridian, and you have just restored circulation in the entire stomach meridian, which starts by the eyes, and ends at your feet. The meridians cross your entire body.

This is the Traditional Chinese Medicine point system. In addition to the main meridians, there are Extra points on the body, which are not located on a meridian, but are useful for specific functions. There are also different acupuncture theories, which use different points.

Locating Acupuncture Points using the Cun

Some points are located by landmarks that are easy to identify, but other points have to be measured to find the location. This is done using the cun system. The cun is a unit of measurement that is about the size of your thumb joint. The reason a cun is used, is because different body sizes require the measurement to be made that is appropriate to the person.

A child, or small adult has different measurements than a tall man. You use the cun measurement of the person you are treating, not your own. You can compare your thumb to their thumb and make an estimate on how much you need to adjust it.

When measuring one cun, you can use your thumb, but for longer measurements you need to use several fingers.

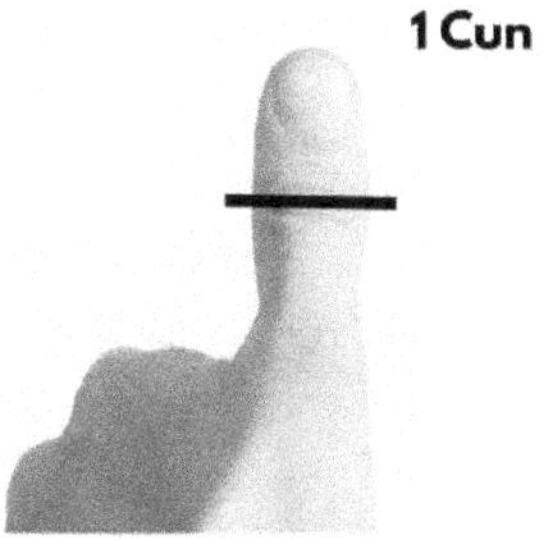

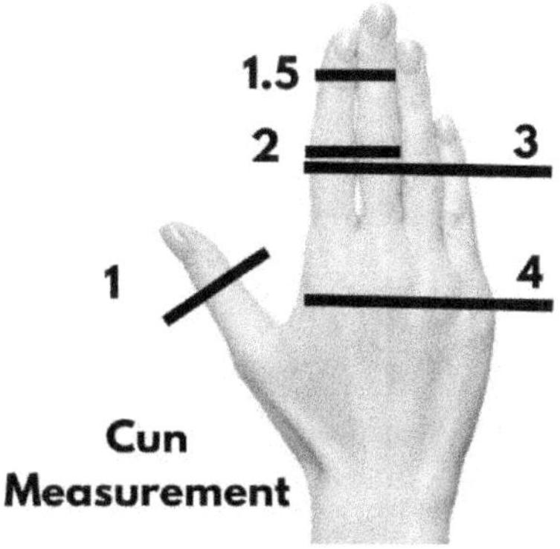

CHAPTER 4

HEAD AND NECK

BRAIN RECOVERY

A stroke disrupts blood flow to the brain, causing oxygen deprivation that kills brain cells within minutes, which can cause permanent damage or long-term disability.

You will most likely get a brain scan, and they might be able to tell you where the stroke occurred. It is not always possible for them to determine that. I'm including brain images. If you know which part of the brain is affected, you can find it on the image.

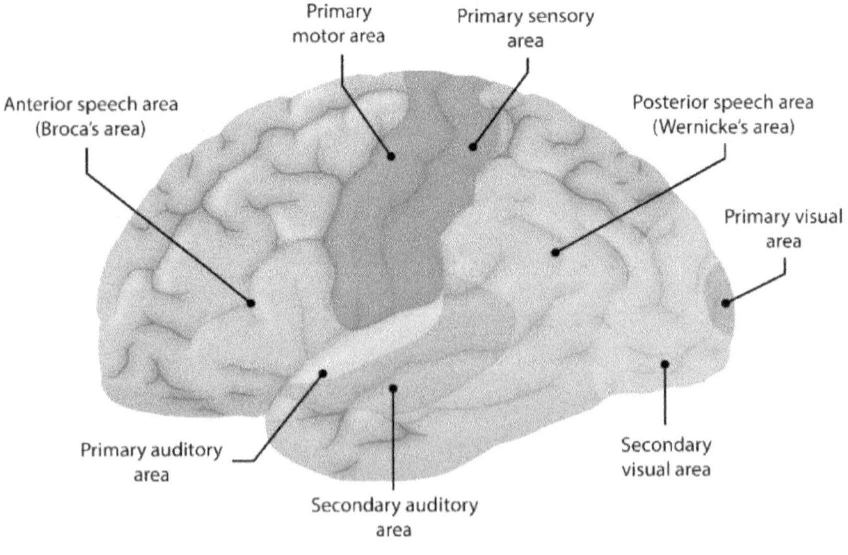

BRAIN FUNCTIONS

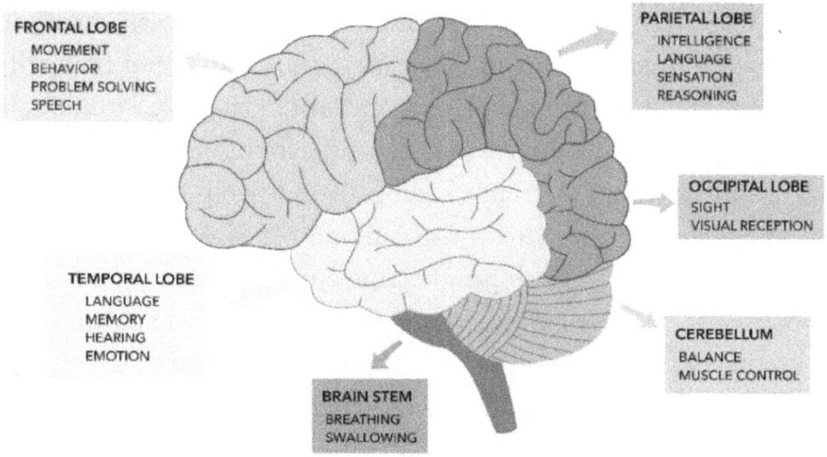

When a person has a stroke, there is damage to the brain. Thrombotic strokes caused by blood clots are the most common. Hemorrhagic strokes are caused by a broken blood vessel. That can be caused by weak blood vessels, please refer to the stroke prevention chapter for information on prevention.

There is damage in the immediate area of the stroke, and an area outside of that, which is called the penumbra. Part of the brain has been damaged, but there is an area around that which can still be recovered. It is inflamed, but there is a chance that area can be healed.

There are numerous acupuncture points to stimulate the brain. Keep in mind that any time you stimulate any point, it sends a signal to the brain.

The first point to treat is Du 20. Du 20 can be located by placing your thumb on the tip of your ear, and the point is at the end of your finger, on the top of your head.

Du 20 benefits the brain, improves concentration, improves memory, treats unconsciousness. I remember using this point on my mom after her stroke, and wondering if it would really work. It seems crazy. I have since found a lot of scientific research that confirms that Du 20 has been proven to help the brain.

After you find Du 20, you can find the Si Shen Cong points, or Four Alert Spirit. Each point is one cun from Du 20, in front of it, behind it, and on either side. These points calm the mind, and help the eyes and ears. They stimulate the brain to improve memory, treat insomnia, dizziness, and eye problems.

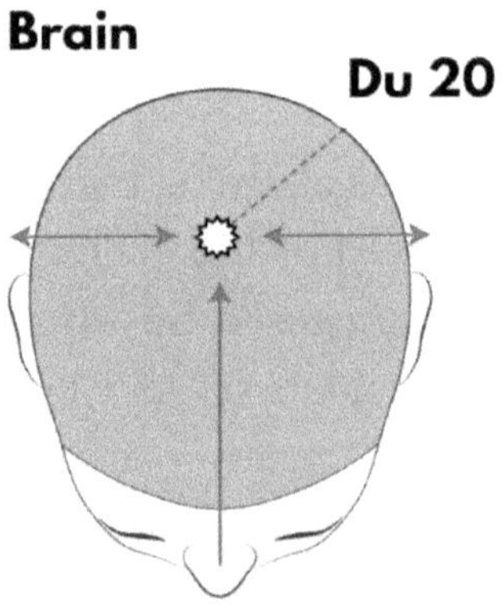

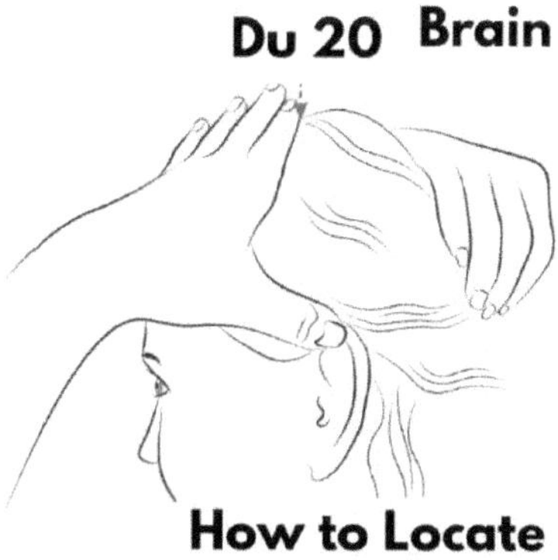

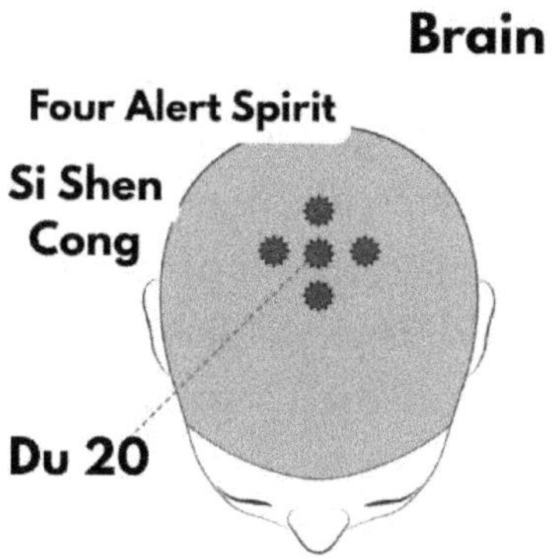

Du 26 is located above the upper lip, on the midline. If you press the tip of your thumbnail just under the nose, you will feel a bone, the point is just below that.

Du 26 is a resuscitation point, it revives consciousness. It also clears the nose, which helps you to distinguish smells, although the best choice for this is Large Intestine 20. Du 26 also treats lockjaw and nosebleeds. It also calms the mind. Press for 3-5 minutes with your thumbnail.

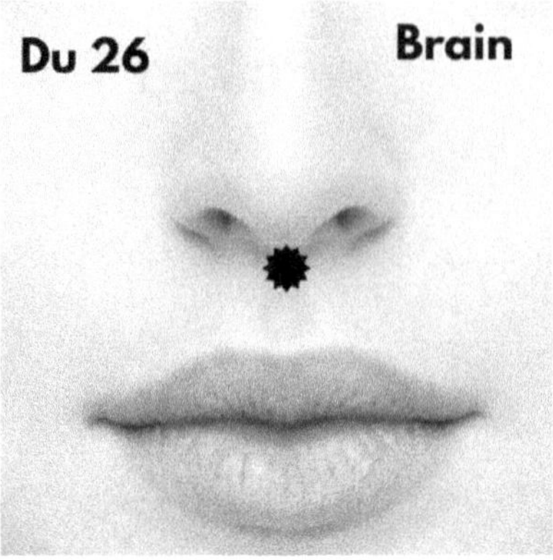

Supplements For Brain Recovery

This is not a complete list of supplements. It is a list of the supplements I found most often in Pubmed research.

It is important to get permission from your doctor before you take any supplement. There is a lot of evidence that supplements can reduce the brain damage that occurs after a stroke, but the medical establishment must have full FDA approval before they can even suggest any supplement.

There might be 100 research articles showing that a supplement benefited stroke patients, but without millions of dollars of research, few doctors will risk their license to administer it. Even if the supplements are already used in the hospital, like NAC, N-acetylcysteine, they cannot just give it to patients unless the hospital and the FDA approve it.

Please be kind to your doctors, nurses, and other hospital staff. They have hard jobs, and must work within the medical system.

DHA and Fish Oil

Fish oil has DHA and EPA. Your brain is about 60% fat. DHA has been shown to reduce the size of the brain damage, and reduce inflammation. It improves focus and memory, and improves mood. I have seen it relieve depression in a couple of days.

Your body needs Omega 3 oils in fish oil. If you are a vegan, there are versions made from algae. I personally take Nordic Naturals DHA, which has a strawberry flavor added. I store mine in the fridge until I'm ready to take it.

If you store Omega 3 oil where it is exposed to heat and light, it can be damaged, and go rancid. That is when it smells fishy, when it is rancid. Do not take stinky fish oil. If it stinks, and causes belching, it is ruined, and it will not help you. Fish oil is very important for brain health.

There is no supplement more important to heal the brain than DHA. The dosage is 3-4 pills, two or three times daily. Everyone should be taking DHA to improve brain function, and prevent dementia.

B Vitamins

Your body needs B vitamins to function normally. Damaged nerves need B vitamins to heal. A good multi vitamin, like Doctor's Best, will have all the vitamins you need. The discount brands are often not the same quality, and type of vitamin and are not absorbed as well.

If you prefer to take a liquid multi vitamin, please be sure that it includes the minerals you need. One brand I found has no minerals like zinc, selenium, magnesium in it. They do not make it clear on the label, which means people think they are getting everything they need.

Benfotiamine is the fat-soluble version of vitamin B 1. It has been used for years to treat nerve damage, and is often recommended for diabetics. Typical benfotiamine dosages range from 150 to 600 mg per day, often for up to 6 months.

For conditions like diabetic neuropathy, a common therapeutic dose is 300 to 600 mg per day. This dosage can be split into two doses of 300 mg each. I have not found any research showing an adverse effect at this dosage.

According to one source because benfotiamine gets converted to thiamine (vitamin B1), and thiamine may cause low blood pressure or low blood glucose, people taking drugs or herbs to lower blood pressure or blood glucose should exercise caution.

In addition to taking B vitamins in a tablet, you can take liquid B 12. It is hard to absorb B 12 in your stomach as you age, and B 12 has been shown to improve brain healing after a stroke. You don't know you are deficient in it until you start taking it and feel a lot better. That is my experience.

Vitamin B 12 has been show to modulate brain damage, and possibly reduce brain inflammation after a stroke. I use Nature's Life B 12. It is methylcobalamin, which is the type you want to take. Cyanocobalamin is not well absorbed, and is not a good option. Some brands are still using cyanocobalamin, because it is cheaper.

Nature's Life liquid B 12 has 5,000 mcg per serving. Some people think they have to get B 12 injections, but you just need to take a high dose supplement, drop it directly in your mouth, and your body absorbs it through the mucosal lining of your mouth. I have personally seen an improvement in my cognitive function after using B 12.

Magnesium and Vitamin C

By most estimates, 80% of people are magnesium deficient. Hospitals often infuse magnesium for patients, but I don't think it is routine for stroke patients. I think it should be considered.

Magnesium is very important for heart and brain health, and without it, you cannot make ATP, which is how your body makes energy. Hospitals normally use magnesium sulphate in intravenous form, to treat other disorders.

Magnesium can also relieve some arrhythmias. I gave my mom magnesium threonate. LivOn Labs makes vitamins that are lyposomal, they are processed with fat, so the vitamin is absorbed better. I also used their Lypo Spheric vitamin C, because I knew that would be absorbed better also. In the beginning she was only allowed to eat pudding, to reduce choke hazard, so I squeezed the vitamins into her pudding.

You do not have to take lyposomal vitamins. They are expensive. If you take vitamin C in a capsule, you can pour the contents into food. I use Reacta C with Bioflavonoids by Solaray. If you take magnesium, please do not take magnesium Oxide. This is not well absorbed. I've read that less than 10% of it is absorbed. It is not what you take, it is what you absorb. Another good magnesium option is Jarrow Mag Mind. That is magnesium threonate. Dr. Sinatra makes a magnesium supplement. It is called Magnesium Broad-Spectrum Complex. It has four types of magnesium. There are many types of magnesium, but that formula is designed for heart patients. Dr. Stephen T. Sinatra has also written a book on treating heart disease, it is called *Reverse Heart Disease Now*.

Magnesium has been shown to reduce infarct volume by up to 60%. That means there will be less brain damage. It helps the brain heal. It reduces heart arrhythmias, and it can help you sleep.

Proteolytic Enzymes

The easiest way to understand how proteolytic enzymes work is to see them as the cleaning crew. Any time you have an injury, or any type of tissue damage, there is damaged tissue that your body has to clean up. The damaged tissue has to be removed, so the blood flow can be restored, and the body can send healing cells into the damaged area, to restore normal function.

Your body naturally makes its own enzymes, but when you are injured, or you are older, your body does not make as much as you need. So, you will heal much slower, because you do not have the resources to clean up the damaged tissue fast enough.

With a stroke, there is the immediate injury to the brain, which needs to be healed, but there is also an area around the damaged area that is deprived of nutrients also. Your body's ability to clean up the damaged tissue, and restore oxygen to the area will be improved by taking enzymes. These enzymes are also used to relieve pain. They not only relieve pain quickly, but they resolve the underlying damaged tissue, so the pain can eventually be completely resolved.

There is also evidence that brain disorders such as Alzheimer's, Parkinsons, and dementia can be improved by taking supplemental enzymes, which helps the body relieve inflammation, which is always present in brain disorders. Inflammation causes scar tissue. The scar tissue might not be visible, but it is there.

Proteolytic enzymes are used to dissolve damaged protein. Take enzymes on an empty stomach, and wait for 30 minutes before you eat. Proteo means protein, and lytic means to break down. Enzymes help to clean out scar tissue, to resolve pain and inflammation, and speed healing. Some people use them to reduce clotting. Blood thinning drugs only prevent future clots. I don't think they clean up tissue that has been damaged.

Enzymes reduce blood clotting, so make sure your doctor approves of your using them. I take Doctor's Best Proteolytic enzymes, because it has several types of enzymes, like nattokinase, and serrapeptase.

Bromelain is another proteolytic enzyme, which is used to treat inflammation, and clean out scar tissue, and relieve pain. This enzyme comes from raw pineapples. You can buy capsules or tablets, or juice a pineapple. Canned pineapple juice has been boiled, and the enzymes are dead. Enzymes are measured in units, like GDU, not milligrams. A good dosage is 2,000 GDU on an empty stomach. Allow 30 minutes for the enzymes to process.

Since enzymes can thin the blood, you should never take them before surgery.

NAC (N-Acetylcysteine)

NAC has been tested extensively to help stroke patients recover. It is one of the top supplements in terms of positive results, which I found on Pubmed.

It is used in hospitals to treat acetaminophen (Tylenol) overdoses. Acetaminophen can damage the liver enough to kill you if you take too much. Hospitals keep NAC in IV form to increase glutathione levels. NAC could be very helpful for stroke treatment. They already know it is safe and effective. But it has not been approved for stroke patients.

"PubMed studies suggest N-acetylcysteine (NAC) acts as a promising, safe, and effective adjunct for stroke treatment by acting as an antioxidant, anti-inflammatory agent, and breaking down thrombi. Research indicates NAC improves neurological outcomes, reduces stroke-induced brain injury, and acts as a thrombolytic agent."

A thrombus is a blood clot. Thrombi are multiple blood clots. There are hundreds of studies showing that NAC is a game changer for stroke patients. It is also used to break down excess mucus in the lungs. It increases glutathione, which is your body's master antioxidant.

NAC is sold over the counter. A common dosage would be 1,500 mg, which is usually 3 capsules. Some people also use it to help recover from Long Covid, because it benefits the immune system, and reduces clotting.

Acupuncture Points Research

In doing research on Pubmed for acupuncture and strokes, I found several articles that researched the use of acupuncture for brain function. It is not necessary for you to know this, I just thought it was interesting, and your doctor or physical therapist might find it interesting also.

Du 26 has been shown to promote an increase in new neurons in the brain cortex. Du 20 and Stomach 36 reduce infarct size in the brain. This reduces damage from the stroke. In one study electroacupuncture was able to inhibit excessive stress, reduce inflammation and promote the repair of neurons, which facilitated healing of ischemic stroke.

BREATHING AND DIAPHRAGM

Diaphragm damage can affect the ability to breathe deeply, and affect the breathing in general. This can also increase the risk for pneumonia.

Ren 14 is located 6 cun above the navel, on the midline. It benefits the diaphragm, opens the chest to improve breathing, and regulates the stomach. It regulates the heart to treat chest pain. It can be used to treat acid reflux, vomiting, and difficulty swallowing.

Ren 17 is located at the fourth intercostal space, which is the area between the ribs. That is how it is defined, but the easiest way to locate it is to use the midpoint between the nipples. If the patient is female, it will be a bit harder to locate. The point is located on the sternum. Don't worry if you do not get the point location exact. Just gently, but firmly press for five minutes. You can massage points above and below the point, in case you feel you might have missed the location. It will all help.

Pericardium 6 is located 2 cun above the wrist crease, between the tendons of the middle of the forearm. This is one of the most important acupuncture points. Pericardium 6 relaxes the diaphragm, and improves chest circulation to treat difficulty breathing. Treat the healthy arm. You can treat both arms.

Pericardium 6 also treats the inability to speak or loss of memory after a stroke. It regulates the heart and stomach and treats nausea, and vomiting. It restores healthy circulation in the chest. It also strengthens and regulates the heart. It is also commonly used to treat anxiety, and insomnia, because it calms the mind. Treat the healthy side.

Ren 12 is not a primary point for the diaphragm, or the lungs, but it regulates circulation in the chest, so I am including it. It is located 4 cun above the navel. Ren 12 treats hiccups, stagnant digestion, and acid reflux. This is a good point to include, because it has a strong regulatory effect on digestion in general.

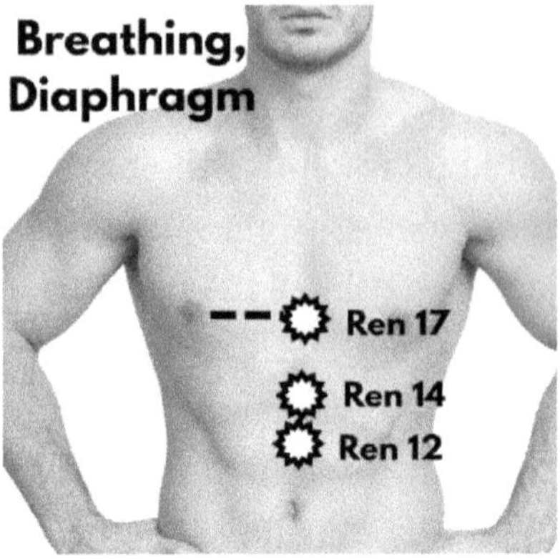

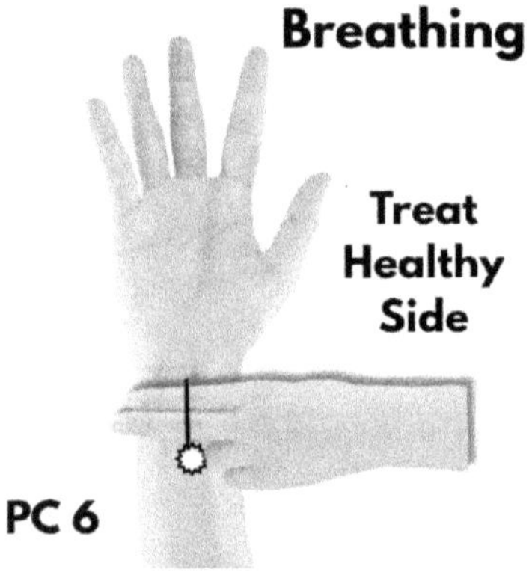

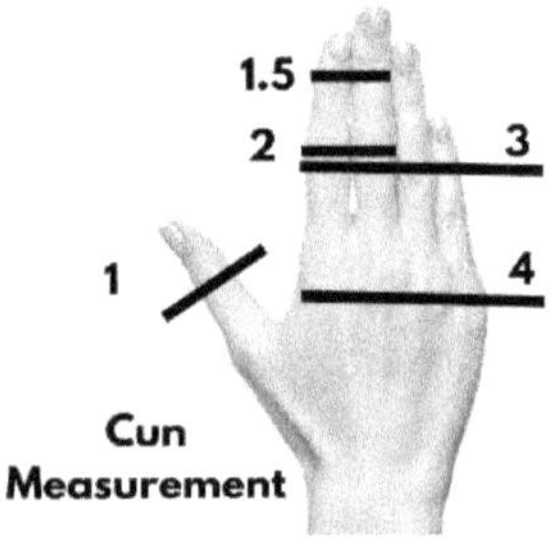

Spine Points – Secondary Points

I doubt you will need to treat points on the spine. I believe the points shown above will be all you need, but I want to include some points on the spine. In case you need them.

The following points are located by the spine, so they might not be easy for you to locate. There is no harm in doing acupressure on all the points in the area. This stimulates the spinal nerves, and will help them to function better. You can just press on and massage the points on the muscles, along the spine, on both sides. That will improve your recovery in general.

Bladder 13 is located 1.5 cun lateral to thoracic vertebrae number 3. This can be located by finding the largest vertebra at the top of the back. That is Cervical 7. Measure counting down from this point. Bladder 13 is the Lung associated point. It regulates and strengthens the lungs. It treats difficult breathing, asthma, and cough.

Bladder 16 is located 1.5 cun lateral to the spine, at the lower border of the sixth thoracic vertebrae. It is used to restore circulation in the chest, treat pericarditis, and diaphragm spasms.

Bladder 17 is located 1.5 cun lateral to the spine, at the lower border of the seventh thoracic vertebra. Bladder 17 is the diaphragm associated point. This means it regulates the diaphragm. It treats hiatal hernia, esophageal constriction, and acid reflux.

Bladder 46 is located 3 cun lateral to T 7.vertebra. Bladder 46 regulates the diaphragm. It treats belching, hiccup, and vomiting.

Stomach 36 is one of the strongest, and most important points on the body. You will already be using this point to restore leg circulation. It has hundreds of potential uses. In the case of a stroke, it is used to treat diaphragm spasms, difficulty swallowing, difficulty breathing, and leg paralysis.

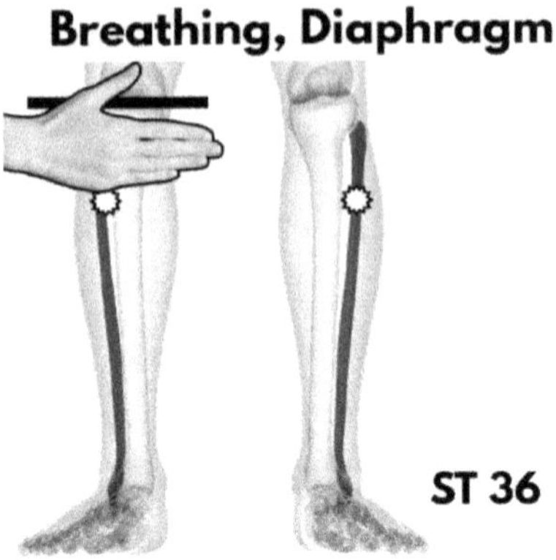

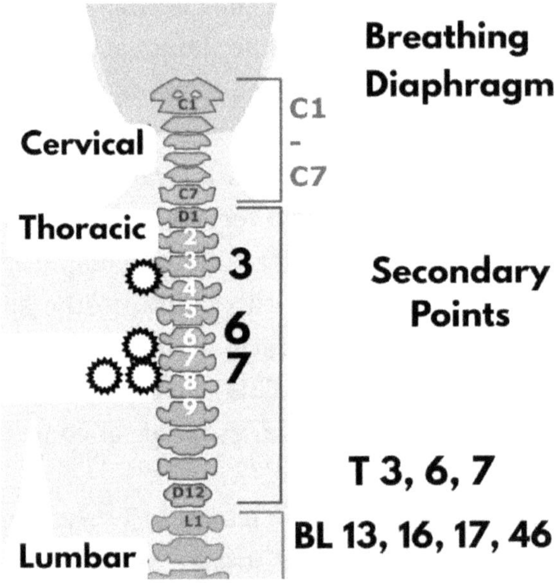

COMA OR LOSS OF CONSCIOUSNESS

There are many acupuncture points that have been used traditionally to restore consciousness in Chinese medicine.

Please be sure to get permission from your medical doctor before you attempt to help someone who is in a coma.

In doing research on this, I found that Du 20, on the top of the head, was the most common point researched. However, Du 26, below the nose, is one of the most commonly used points, according to Chinese medicine literature. I would start at the top of the head first, then work my way down, stimulating each point about five minutes.

Each time you do acupressure, you are increasing the ability of the patient to recover. It is a series of treatments. There is no way to know how long it will take, or if it will work, but it is worth trying.

Locked-in syndrome can also be treated with the points in this chapter. Locked in means that the patient is aware, but cannot move or speak. A brain stem injury is the most common cause of this syndrome. I am not an expert in comas or unconsciousness, so please speak with your doctor about this.

Coma Explained

A coma, or loss of consciousness is when someone has minimal brain activity, cannot be woken up, and cannot react to anything in the environment. There are different levels of a coma. A severe coma will not be able to open the eyes or respond to sound, pain, or touch. The sleep-wake cycle is disrupted.

A coma from a stroke rarely lasts longer than four weeks. People in a coma are sometimes aware of what is going on around them, but they cannot respond. I would assume the patient could hear you, and explain what you are doing, and offer positive words.

Hemorrhagic strokes, which are caused by a burst blood vessel, are more likely to cause a coma. About 17% of people who have a hemorrhagic stroke suffer from a coma. Only 3% of patients with ischemic, or blood clot strokes, suffer from a coma.

Stroke patients usually regain consciousness slowly, by moving through coma recovery stages.

Acupressure Points

Du 20 is located on the top of the head. To find this point, place the tip of your thumb on the tip of your ears. Your fingertips usually land on Du 20. The Du meridian is pronounced Doo, and it is also called the Governing Vessel. It corresponds to the spine. After you locate the area of Du 20, you can verify that you are on the midline, by running your finger from your nose, up to the top of your head.

Du 20 has many functions, but the ones related to stroke are: Improves concentration, revives consciousness, and it treats rectal and uterine prolapse. It improves blood flow to the brain, and helps to restore brain function. Du 20 is a top point to treat many stroke issues, because it revives the brain.

Du 26 is located on the upper lip. It is just below the nose. If you run your thumb along the area below your nose, you should feel a dip in the bone. The point is below that. Du 26 treats coma, lockjaw, nosebleeds, and the inability to distinguish smells. It is a resuscitation point, and it revives consciousness. To activate this point, I would use the tip of the thumbnail, pointed upward toward the nose. Put the tip of your thumbnail under the dip in the bone. Press for five minutes.

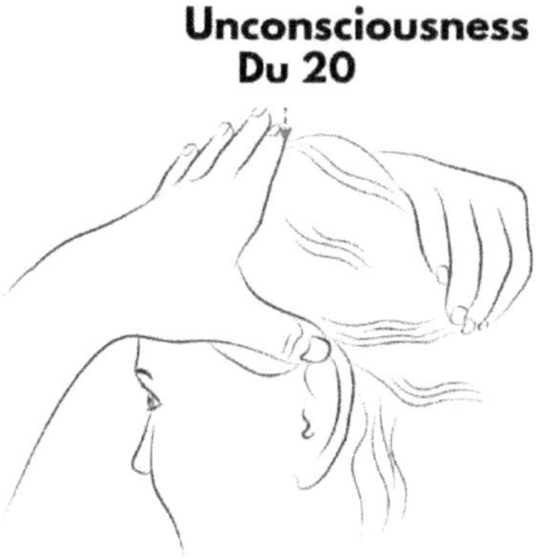
Unconsciousness
Du 20

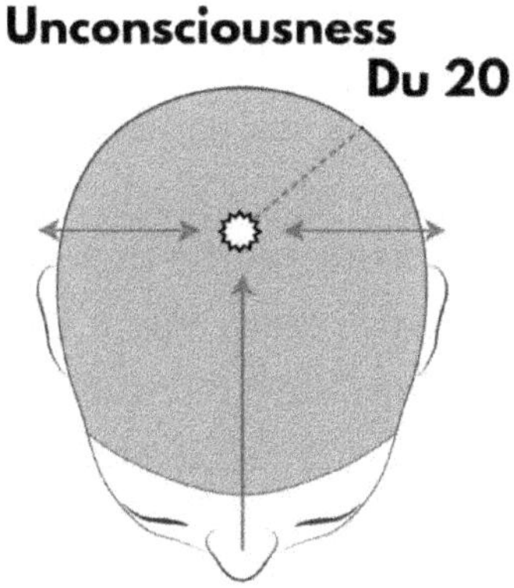
Unconsciousness
Du 20

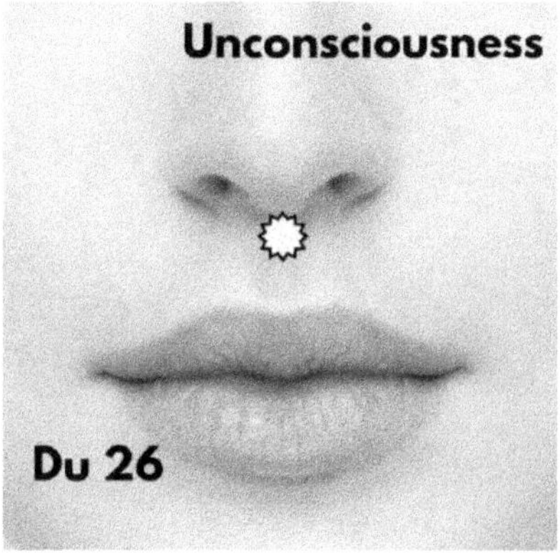
Unconsciousness
Du 26

Finger Resuscitation Points

Acupressure points on the fingers can be activated easily by pressing the tip of the fingernail into the points. Press for 5 minutes per point.

Heart 9 is located .1 cun behind the corner of the nail on the little finger. It revives consciousness, regulates the heart, and calms the mind.

Large Intestine 1 is located on the index finger, .1 cun from the corner of the nail. It revives consciousness, and relieves throat pain by moistening the throat.

Small Intestine 1 is located on the little finger, .1 cun from the corner of the nail. It treats loss of consciousness after a stroke.

Pericardium 8 is located on the palm, between the second and third hand bones. The end of the middle fingertip will land on the point on the palm, when the fingers are bent.

Pericardium 9 is located on the tip of the middle finger. It restores consciousness, and some sources say it restores the ability to speak after a stroke.

Unconsciousness

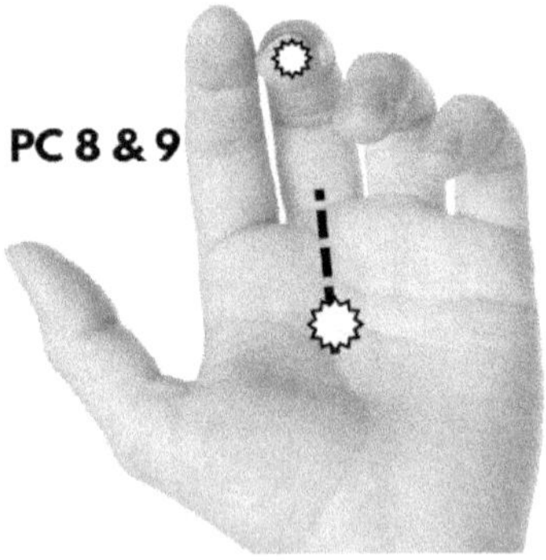

Unconsciousness

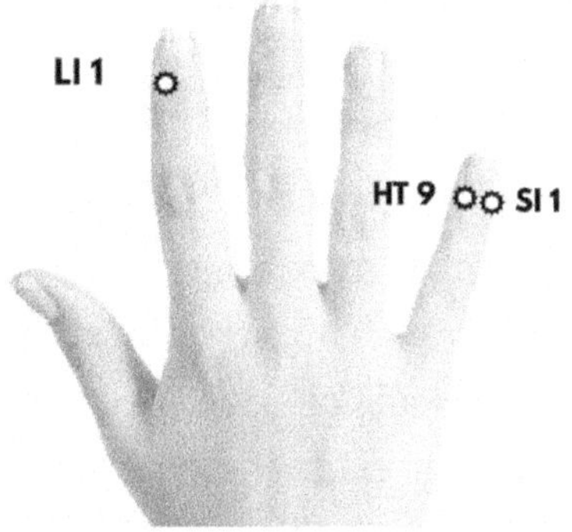

Unconsciousness

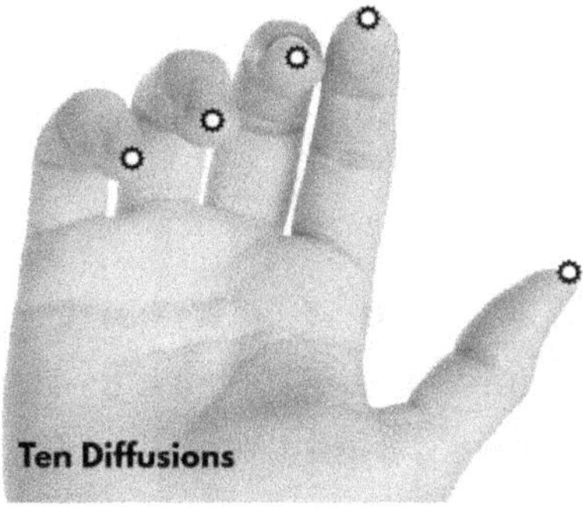

Fingertip Points

The Ten Diffusions are extra points, they are not located on meridians, so they are not numbered, but called by name. In Chinese it is Shi Xuan. I will list it as Ten Diffusions. These points are on the tips of the ten fingers, about .1 cun from the fingernail. They revive consciousness, and help with stroke recovery.

You can activate the points with the tip of a fingernail. The points are just under the end of the fingernail, and they are very sensitive. Press firmly for 3-5 minutes. I would treat both hands. You could also use a lancet, which is used by diabetics, and easy to find. Some people elicit a small drop of blood from these points. This is a classical usage in Chinese medicine.

Abdomen Points

Ren 4, 6, and 8 are on the abdomen. These points are traditionally treated with moxibustion. This is burning the Mugwort herb over the area. This strongly strengthens the body.

Moxa is not practical for most people. You can use a hot water bottle, or heating pad instead. Be careful with the temperature to avoid burns. All you need is a gentle heat to stimulate the points. You do not have to apply heat, but it is an option. You can simply press very firmly on each point for about five minutes and see what results you get. Warming the area will improve circulation in the area.

Practical Treatment

Ren 4 is located 3 cun below the navel, on the midline. It strengthens the kidneys, and uterus. It treats urinary incontinence, and urinary retention. It also treats organ prolapse, such as uterine, or rectal prolapse.

Ren 6 is located 1.5 cun below the navel, on the midline. It restores collapsed yin or yang, regulates urination, treats uterine prolapse, and strengthens the kidneys. To locate this point, just measure down from the navel, using two fingers. Press firmly, and massage gently to activate the point.

Ren 8 is located on the navel. Ren 8 restores consciousness with moxibustion. Do not press on this point. It is only treated with heat. I have removed this point from the image, in case people don't read the text.

Unconsciousness

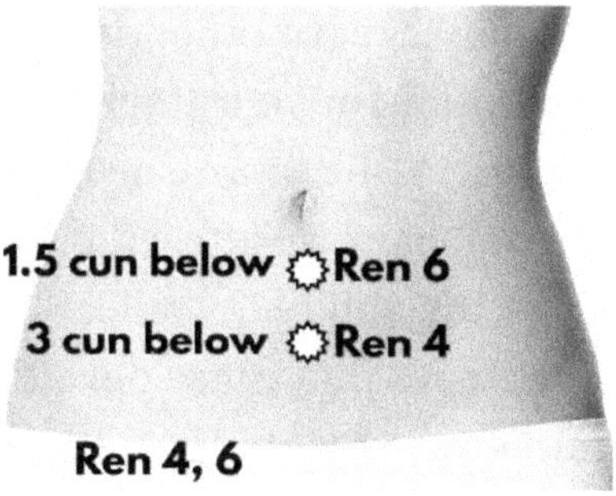

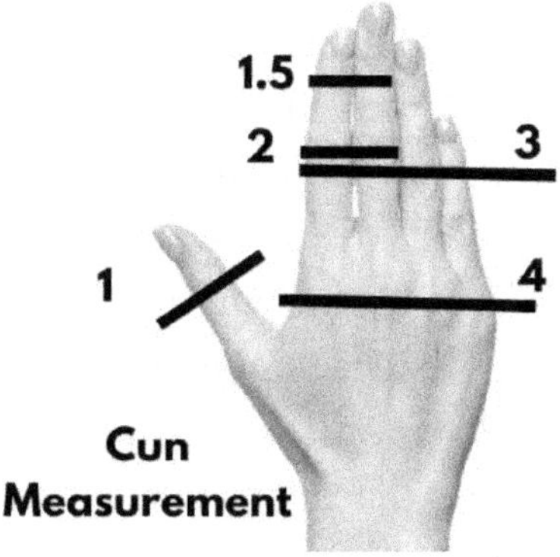

DEVIATED EYE AND FACE

Please do not use any massager or other device around your eyes. Ear seeds are the best option, or your fingertip.

A stroke can affect the face causing muscle weakness, drooping, and paralysis. It can also affect the eyelid, cheek, mouth, or tongue. It may affect the ability to smile. Slurred speech might be caused by the same issues that cause deviation.

There are numerous points that can help, starting with Large Intestine 20. Large Intestine 20 is located at the naso-labial groove, at the level of the midpoint of the lateral border of the nostril. It treats loss of sense of smell, mouth deviation, nosebleeds, and trigeminal neuralgia.

Treat the affected side after a stroke. If it has been a few months since your stroke, treat both sides, to balance your face.

Ren 24 is located in the center of the mento-labial groove. This is located between the chin and lips, in the middle. Ren 24 relaxes the tendons in the face, and can be used to treat deviation of the mouth and eye, lockjaw, and facial paralysis.

Jia Cheng Jian – Adjacent to Container of Fluids is located 1 cun lateral to Ren 24, on both sides of the face. This point treats deviation of the mouth and eye. It also treats facial paralysis, and trigeminal neuralgia.

Small intestine 18 is located directly below the outer edge of the eye, in the depression at the lower border of the cheek bone. It treats facial paralysis, trigeminal neuralgia, deviated eye and mouth, eyelid twitching, and cheek swelling.

Tai Yang, which could be translated as Supreme Yang, is located about 1 cun, or thumb width, behind the midpoint between the lateral end of the eyebrow and the outer canthus. I know that sounds confusing. With acupressure you should not miss it. This point also treats vision problems.

Stomach 3 is located directly below the pupil, at the level of the lower border of the nostrils. It treats facial paralysis, trigeminal neuralgia, eyelid twitching, excess tear production, and swelling of the lips and cheeks.

Stomach 4 is located .4 cun lateral to the corner of the mouth. It treats facial paralysis, trigeminal neuralgia, excessive saliva production, drooling, deviation of the mouth, toothache, eyelid twitching, and inability to close the eye.

Pericardium 5 is located 3 cun above the wrist crease, between the tendons. It strengthens the hear, and treats drooling caused by a stroke.

Eye Deviation

Eye deviation is when the eyes do not point in the same direction. This is caused by the muscles that control eye movement not working properly. After a stroke, the muscles of the eyes can be affected in the same way that the muscles of the arms and legs are.

Acupuncture treats this by stimulating points around the eyes that stimulate blood flow and regulate energy circulation. Many of the points that treat mouth deviation and facial paralysis, also treat eye deviation. I suggest you just treat all the points, as there is no downside, and you might not be able to tell for sure that you can rule out that problem. If you just stimulate the points, you are helping to restore function to the whole face.

Some of the points I am suggesting for eye deviation, do not specifically have the indication of eye deviation, such as Bladder 2. But every person is different, and you might need a few extra points.

Do Not Use any Massager by Your Eyes

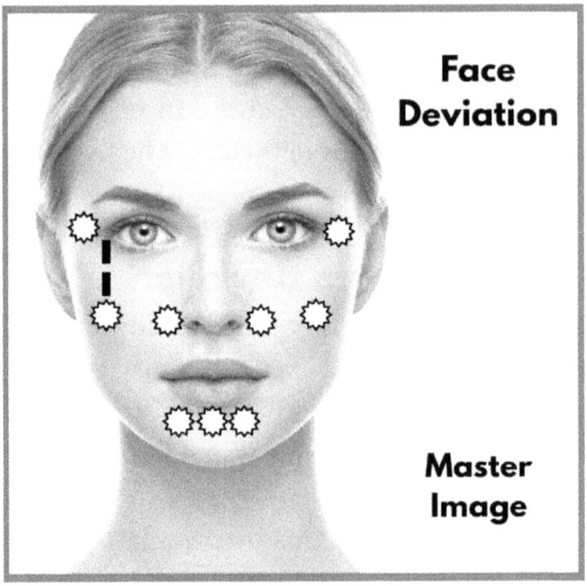

Do Not Use Any Massage Device by Eyes

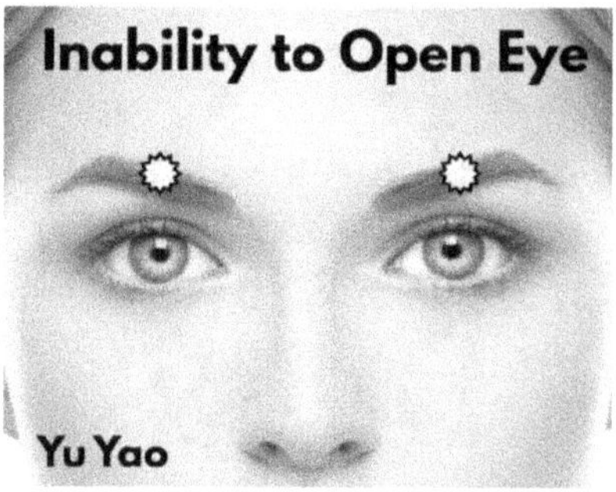

Eye Opening, Closing Eye Muscles

Do Not Use Any Massage Device by Eyes

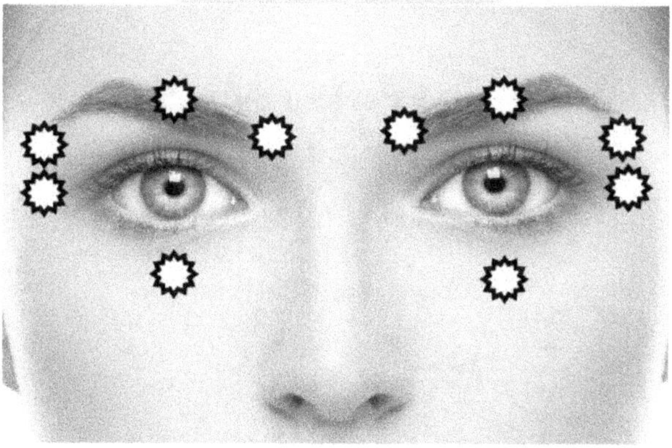

Ability to Close Eye

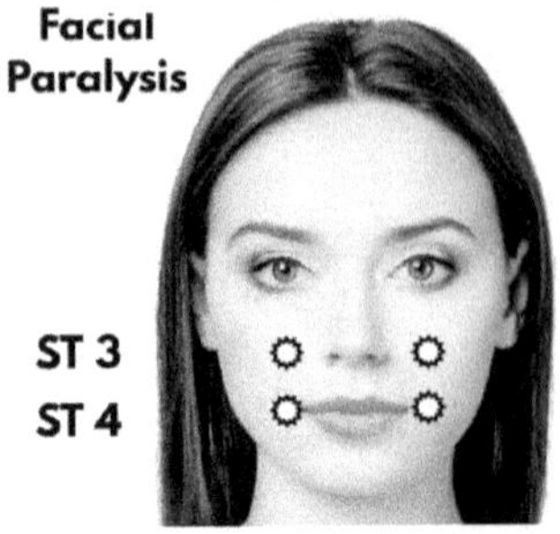

Drooling

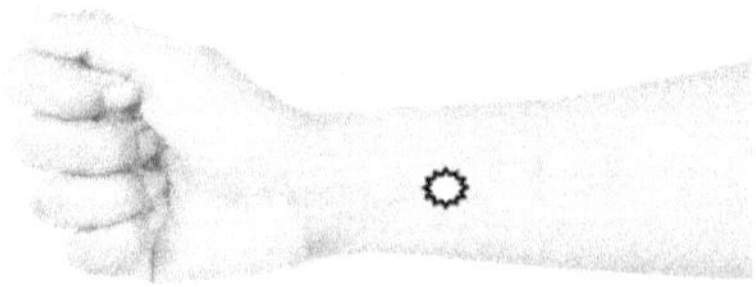

Pericardium 5

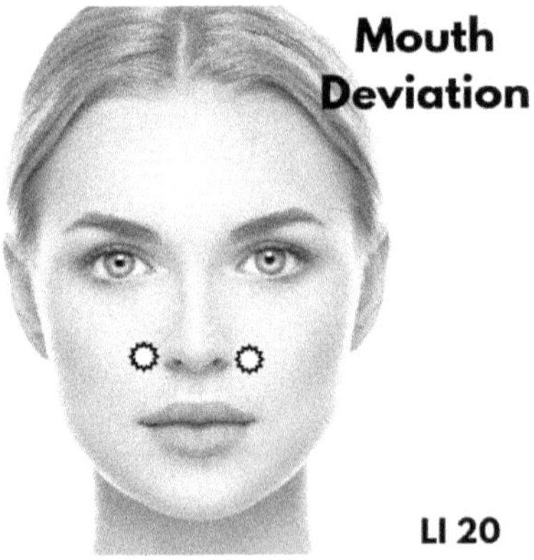

Deviated Eye & Mouth

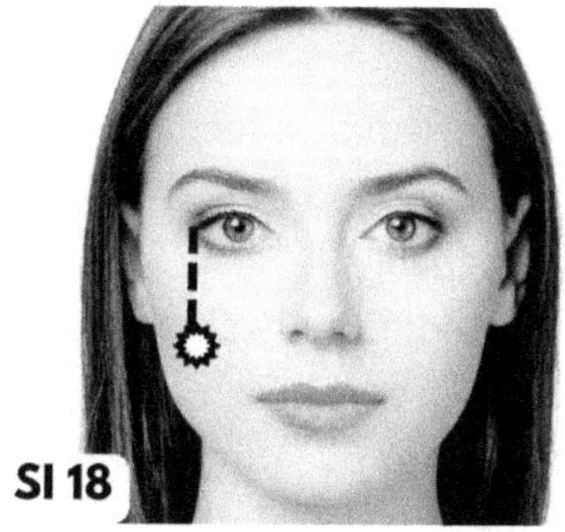

Eye Deviation

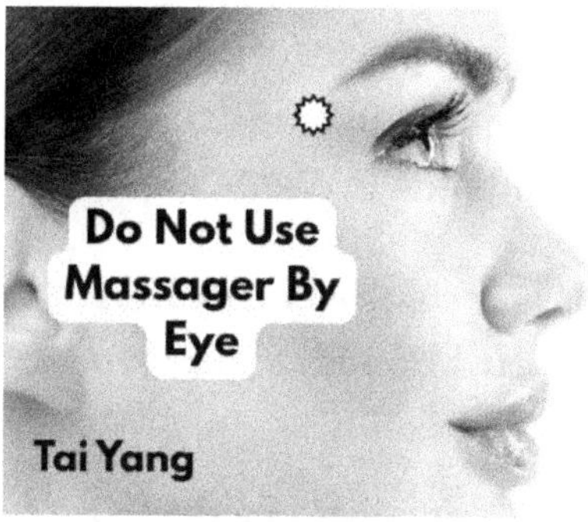

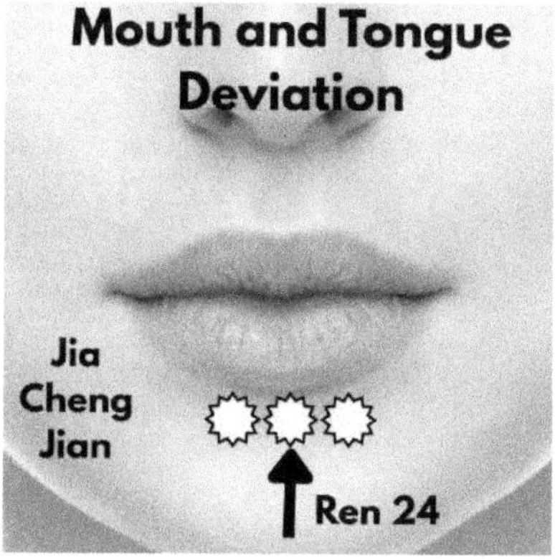

DROOPING EYELIDS

The nerves around the eye can be affected by a stroke. The muscle that lifts the eyelid can be treated by activating the point called Yu Yao, or Fish Waist in English.

The point is located directly above the pupil of the eye, in the middle of the eyebrow.

Press firmly for about five minutes. Make sure to look in a mirror when you do this, as your ability to feel can be affected by the stroke. Look in a mirror, and press gently. You can also use ear seeds, but do not use a massage device.

This point is very popular for facial acupuncture. It treats drooping eyelids, which can also be caused by tight muscles. It treats the muscle that lifts the eyelid.

Drooping Eyelids

Do Not Use Massager

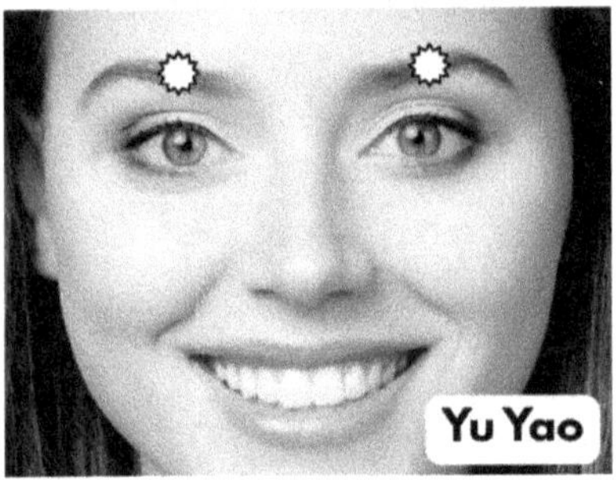

HEARING

There are several points by the ear that stimulate circulation in the ear. These points can be used for hearing loss due to any cause.

Gallbladder 2 is located in front of the ear. It is described as in front of the intertragic notch, on the posterior border of the condyloid process of the mandible. I think you would agree, that is easier to just look at a picture of the point.

Gallbladder 2 opens the ears to treat deafness, tinnitus, ear infections, and it treats ear pain. It also treats jaw pain, and TMJ pain.

Small Intestine 19 is located just above Gallbladder 2. It treats deafness, ear inflammation, tinnitus, and vertigo due to ear problems.

Triple Burner 21 is located above Small Intestine 19. It opens and regulates the ears. It restores normal circulation in the ears. It treats tinnitus, deafness, and earache.

Triple Burner 17 is located behind the earlobe, between the mandible and mastoid process. It treats deafness, itching inside the ear, earache, tinnitus, lockjaw, and dimness of vision.

Gallbladder 20 is located in the hollow between the sternocleidomastoid and trapezius muscles, at the base of the skull.

Gallbladder 20 treats blurred vision, dizziness, headaches, migraines, neck pain, and shoulder pain. It improves circulation to the eyes, and treats loss of speech after a stroke. Gallbladder 20 also opens blocked ears. This point has dozens of functions that help you recover from a stroke.

I would use ear seeds on the points by the ear, because the nerves are very sensitive to stimulation.

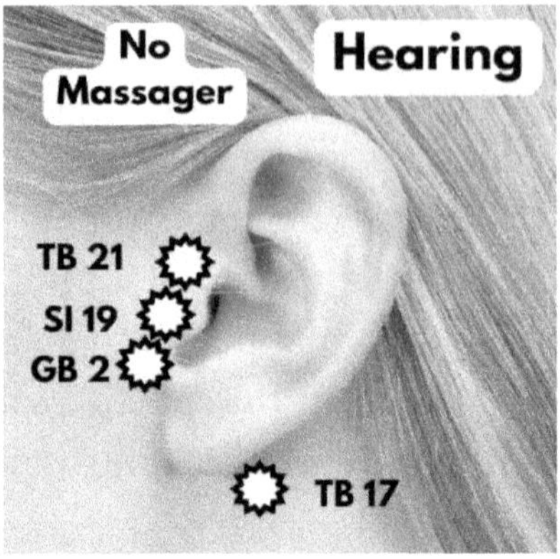

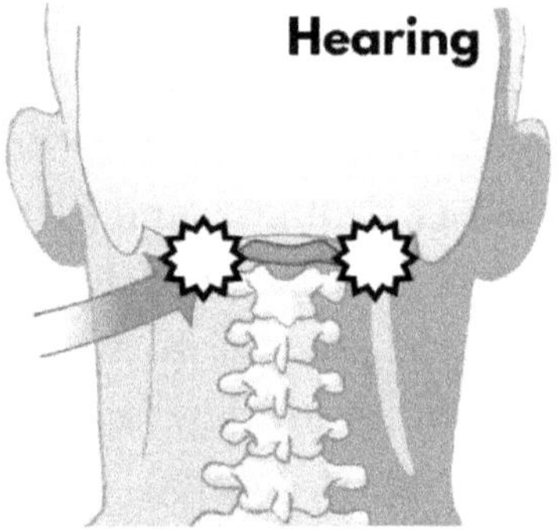

Gallbladder 20

HICCUPS

Hiccups are caused by involuntary spasms of the diaphragm muscle, followed by a fast closure of the vocal cords.

Ren 12 is the first point to treat. It is one hand width above the navel, on the midline of the front of the body. Press firmly for about five minutes, you can massage the point into the muscle. It might ache a little.

After you treat Ren 12, just work your way up the abdomen, one point at a time. Treating several points on this meridian will make the effect much stronger.

Ren 12 is a major point for any stomach issue. It regulates the stomach, descends stomach energy, which means that if you are vomiting, or your esophagus is not functioning correctly, Ren 12 will regulate it and make it work normally. It treats hiccups, acid reflux, and regulates stomach function.

Ren 13 is 5 cun above the navel, on the midline, above Ren 12. It also treats acid reflux and regulates the stomach, like Ren 12. It also treats nausea, and gastritis, which is called stomach fire in Chinese medicine. It is a burning sensation in your stomach.

Ren 14 is 6 cun above the navel, on the midline. It benefits the diaphragm, opens the chest, and regulates the stomach and heart. It also treats difficulty swallowing.

Ren 17 is at the fourth intercostal space, which is the space between the ribs. It is at the level of the nipples, which is easier to find on men than women. Ren 17 treats diaphragm spasms, difficulty swallowing, esophageal constriction, hiccups, and wheezing.

Pericardium 6 is 2 cun above the wrist crease, between the tendons on the middle of the forearm. Be sure to hold your hand level, or flat with the same level as the arm. Do not bend your hand back, because that changes the measurement.

Pericardium 6 is famous for treating nausea from morning sickness. Pericardium 6 has many functions. The most important functions for this book are hiccups, inability to speak or loss of memory after a stroke, insomnia, nausea, palpitations, and heart rhythm disorders, such as atrial fibrillation. It regulates the heart, and restores healthy circulation in the chest. For heart arrythmias, it should be combined with Heart 5, and 7.

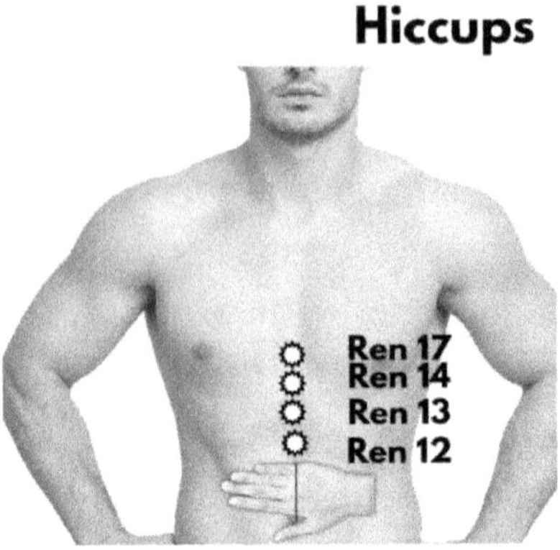

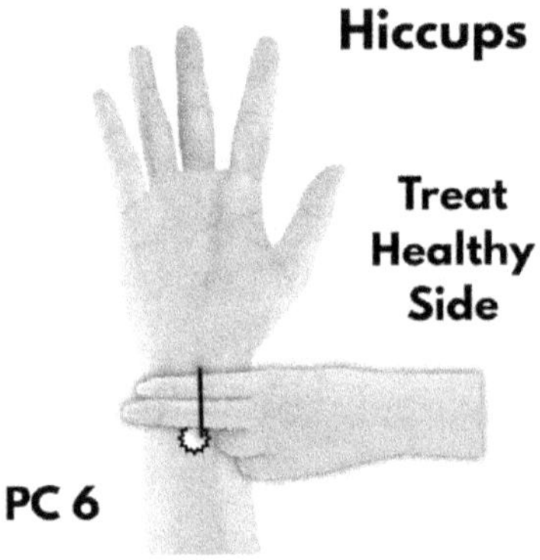

LOCKJAW

Lockjaw, or tight jaw muscles, can restrict the ability to open the mouth. You might also have jaw spasms. These issues can affect your ability to swallow or speak.

Du 26 is above the upper lip, on the midline. Divide the distance between the top of the upper lip, and the border of the nose into thirds. This point is located at the upper third part. I like to use the tip of my thumbnail to press on that point. You will feel a little notch under the bone.

Du 26 treats the inability to distinguish smells, coma, lockjaw, muscle spasms, nosebleeds, and it revives consciousness after fainting, or a stroke.

Ren 24 is located in the depression in the center of the mento-labial groove. Translation: located between the chin and lips, in the middle. Ren 24 relaxes the tendons in the face. It treats deviation of the mouth and eye, lockjaw, facial paralysis, and neck pain.

Stomach 4 is located .4 cun lateral to the corner of the mouth. It treats facial paralysis, excessive saliva production, deviation of the mouth, eyelid twitching, and inability to close the eye. It also treats trigeminal neuralgia.

Stomach 5 is located in front of the angle of the jaw, in front of the masseter muscle. It treats Facial paralysis, facial pain and swelling, lockjaw, mouth deviation, and toothache.

Stomach 6 is located one finger width in front of and above the lower angle of the mandible, which is the jaw bone. It treats facial paralysis, jaw tension, and TMJ. It clears blockages in the meridian that can be caused by a stroke, or regular jaw clenching. It treats difficulty opening the mouth.

Stomach 7 is located at the lower border of the cheekbone, in the depression in front of the condyloid process of the jawbone.

If you walk your fingers along your jawbone toward your ear, you will feel it. Stomach 7 treats lockjaw, or difficulty opening the mouth, facial paralysis, jaw dislocation, tinnitus, TMJ, and deafness.

Triple Warmer 17 is located behind the earlobe, between the jawbone and the mastoid process of the skull. This is a little lump in that area. It benefits the ears, treats deafness, tinnitus, lockjaw, and dimness of vision.

Small Intestine 18 is located directly below the outer edge of the eye, in the depression at the lower border of the cheekbone. It treats facial paralysis, trigeminal neuralgia, deviated eye and mouth, eyelid twitching, and cheek swelling.

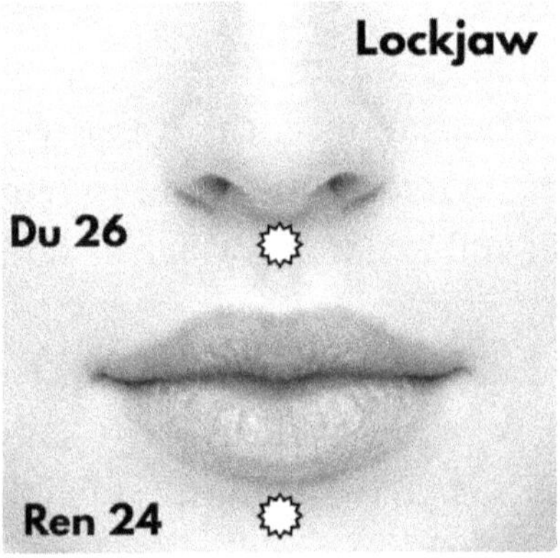

Do Not Use any Massager by Your Eyes or Ears

Lockjaw

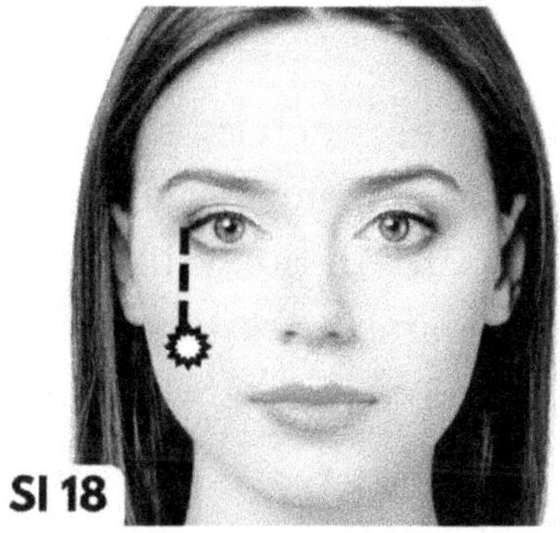
SI 18

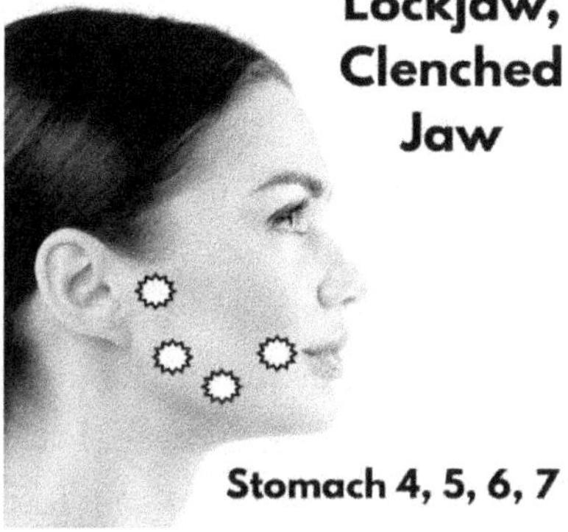
Lockjaw,
Clenched
Jaw
Stomach 4, 5, 6, 7

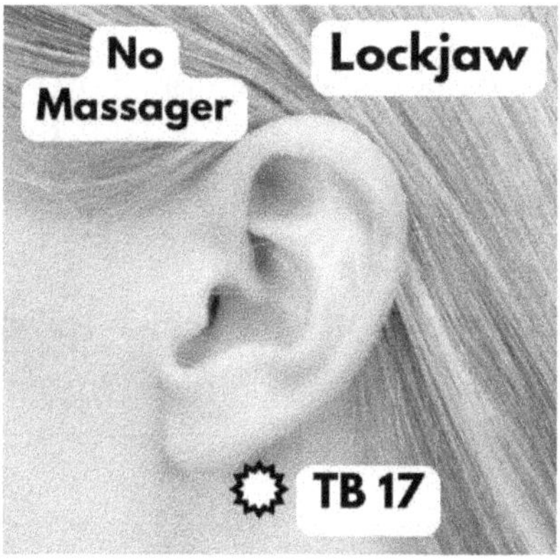
No
Massager
Lockjaw
TB 17

SMELL AND TASTE

About 95% of the ability to taste, is determined by the ability to smell, or distinguish smells. So restoring the ability to smell should restore the ability to taste. In the unlikely event that you still have the inability to taste, after treating the ability to smell, please refer to the speaking chapter to see which points treat the tongue.

A patient of mine had lost the ability to smell, due to chronic sinus infections and allergies. After taking Chinese herbs, and getting acupuncture, his chronic sinus infections went away, and he was able to smell again. This point can also help the ability to smell if the olfactory nerve is damaged by viruses or bacteria.

There is only one point you need to treat to restore the ability to smell, and that is Large Intestine 20. The location is at the midpoint of the lateral border of the nostrils. I would treat both sides. Just press firmly, until you feel the cheek bone. Press firmly for five minutes on both sides. You can also use a mini massager on this point.

Large Intestine 20 treats the loss of sense of smell, mouth deviation from Bell's Palsy, or other nerve problems, nosebleeds, sinus headaches, trigeminal neuralgia, and it opens the sinuses. Acupuncture points excel at treating nerve issues, because the points help to restore healthy circulation.

The olfactory nerve is located inside the sinuses. This gives you the ability to process smells. I believe Large Intestine 20 helps to restore the function of this nerve.

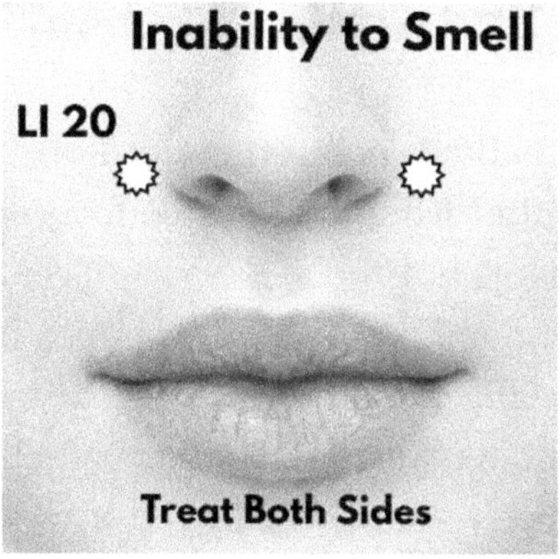
Inability to Smell
LI 20
Treat Both Sides

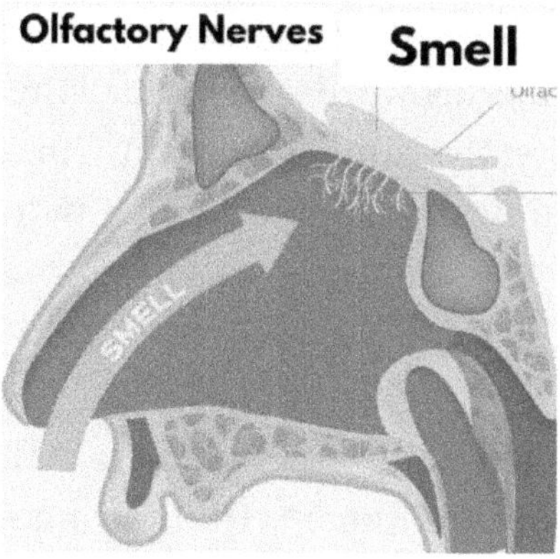
Olfactory Nerves
Smell
SMELL

SPEAKING, APHASIA

Poststroke aphasia affects about one third of stroke patients, and 30-43% of them suffer from long term effects of aphasia.
The ability to speak is not the same as aphasia. Aphasia includes language processing ability, and other issues in communication. Since there is a feedback loop, I believe that treating the parts of the body that regulate speaking should be helpful to restore the part of the brain that was affected by the stroke.

Speaking requires the coordination of approximately **70 to over 100 muscles**. These muscles work together in the chest, neck, jaw, tongue, lips, and larynx to produce sound, regulate breathing, and articulating words. So treat all the areas as often as you need, until you get the results you want. This can be one of the more complicated things to treat, with a lot more points needing treatment.

The points in this chapter are to treat the tongue and mouth.

There are many point options to treat this problem. The most important points are Ren 23, Du 15, Du 20, and Jin Jin, Yu Ye.

The points closer to, or on the tongue muscle itself, on the neck, are the first ones to try. To restore the ability to speak, you need to address the tongue, but you might also need to treat facial muscles that are not working correctly after the stroke.

I am starting with the most important points, and moving down to points you can use if the first points are not enough. Do not give up. It might take 5-10 treatments to notice a difference. Your goal is to stimulate these points, which makes the brain recognize the area again. These points will work if you activate them enough.

It Is Working, Keep Pressing

Press firmly for five minutes minimum. You might **feel** like you are not getting results, but your body is processing the points. You might feel a difference in an hour, 6 hours, or the next day. You never know how long it will take for acupuncture or acupressure to work. Just don't give up.

The ability to speak well can be affected by face muscles, and the tongue muscle itself. Everyone is different. Please refer to the eye and mouth deviation chapters for facial muscle points.

Treating Ren 23 and Points Around It

Ren 23 is located above the Adam's apple, in the depression of the upper border of the hyoid bone. This point is very tender, and many of the muscles of the tongue attach to this bone.

There are alternative areas under the jaw, which might also be helpful. It is hard to know exactly which nerves and muscles are affected, so I would do acupressure on the whole area, on the meridians and points as shown. Treat each point a few minutes. Be gentle in this area.

To treat Ren 23, I would press my thumb underneath the jawbone, holding onto the jaw. This gives you better leverage to press firmly enough. I would start pressing right under the jawbone, then move my way down lower, towards the root of the tongue. It is not very far from the jawbone. The image showing the hyoid bone makes it look like it is further down the neck, that is the only way to show the bone and anatomy. If you do not stretch your neck out, like in the image, the points are closer to the jawbone.

Ren 23 is called Lian Quan in Chinese. On either side of Ren 23 are extra points, called Jia Lian Quan. They should all be treated. That is the root of the tongue. If you use a massager in this area, be careful. It is very sensitive. You do not need strong stimulation to make it work. You can also try ear seeds.

Please remember that you might not be able to feel anything at first, and pressing too hard could cause pain. Be gentle.

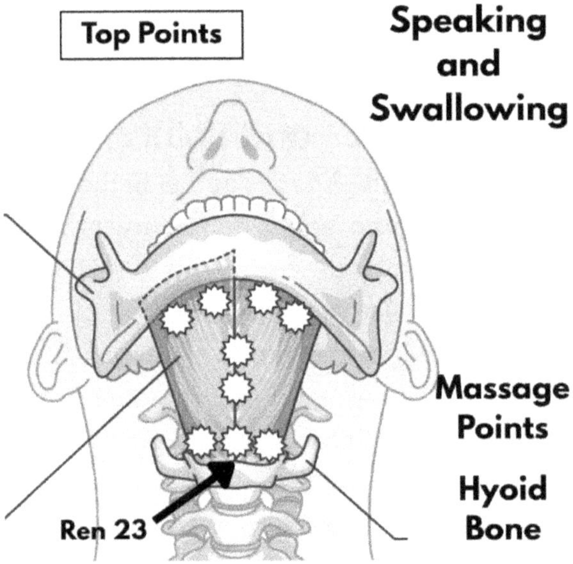

Du 20 is located at the top of the head. Place your thumbs on the tip of your ears, and where your fingers touch should be the midline. Du 20 is very important. It might not seem like it, but Du 20 has been proven to improve brain function. It improves concentration, and memory. It revives consciousness, restores collapsed energy in the body. The Du meridian is pronounced (Doo).

Du 20 is one of the most commonly used points to treat stroke patients in all the studies I found. Be sure to locate the point on the midline, in the center of the body. Double check from the nose to make sure it is centered.

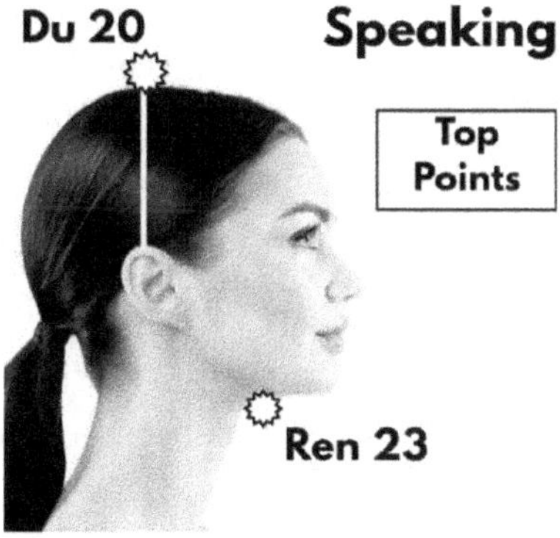

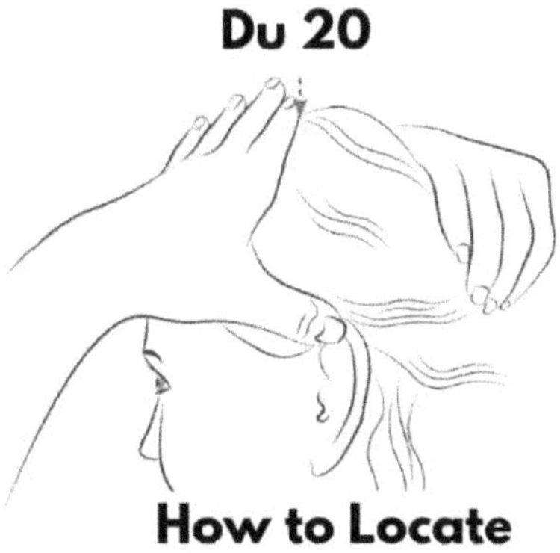

Du 15 is located one half cun above the posterior hairline, below the spinous process of cervical vertebra one, or C 1. It is located opposite the root of the tongue. Du 15 treats the inability to speak after a stroke, tongue stiffness, and neck pain.

There are points located underneath the tongue. I was not even aware of them until I started doing research on how to treat strokes with acupuncture. They consistently show up in scientific literature on how to restore the ability to speak with acupuncture. The points are located under the tongue muscle, not on the muscle. They are treated in different ways. Some people insert needles, others do bloodletting.

Gallbladder 20 is at the base of the back of the skull. It is located between the sternocleidomastoid and trapezius muscles. The indentation there is very small, so don't worry about getting it perfect. When you are doing acupressure, the fingers, or the mini massager will cover a large area, and that's OK. Gallbladder 20 has many functions to help you recover from a stroke.

Gallbladder 20 treats blurred vision, dizziness, and it opens blocked ears. It treats migraines, and loss of speech after a stroke.

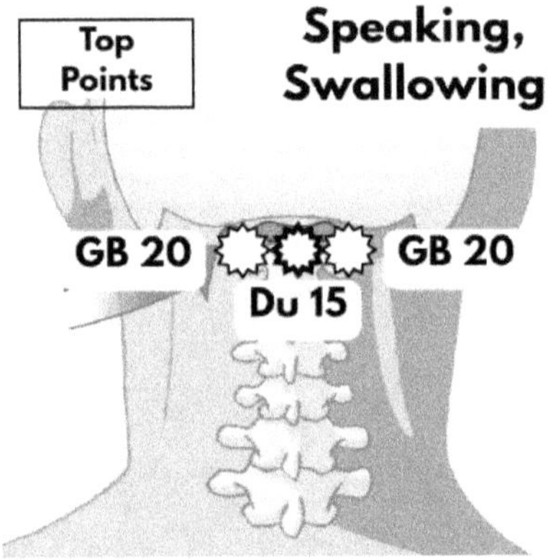

Heart 5 is located 1 cun above the wrist crease, on the thumb side of the flexor carpi tendon, which is easy to find if you move your little finger. This tendon is large and moves up and down when you move your little finger. Measure one cun by using your thumb, placing it on the wrist crease.

Heart 5 regulates the heart rhythm, so it will help with atrial fibrillation and other heart arrhythmias. It treats palpitations, which is when you feel your heart beating. This might or might not be caused by an issue with the heart itself.

In Chinese medicine, the heart energy can become weak over time, and herbal tonics can be given that strengthen the heart and relieve palpitations and insomnia.

Heart 5 treats sudden loss of voice, with tongue stiffness. I typically combine heart 7 and heart 5 together. Heart 7 is located on the wrist crease, and Heart 5 is located one cun above it.

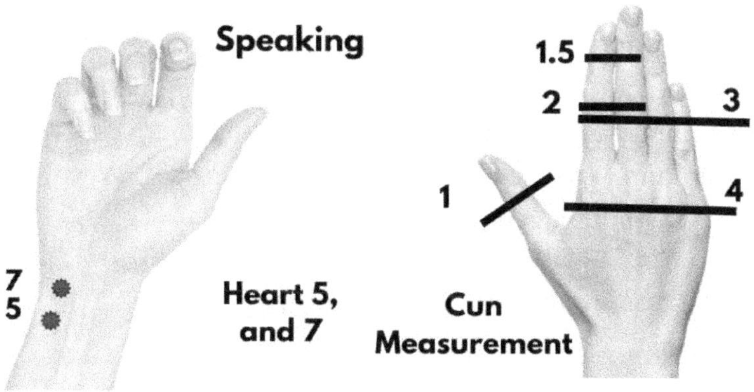

Research on Heart 5 and Heart 7 Effects on The Brain

Your doctor or physical therapist might be more interested in a little information I found on the confirmation of how these acupuncture points help. This was not all the research I found confirming what Chinese medicine has known about how the points work to treat different issues.

Right side Heart 5 activates multiple language related brain regions such as the left insula, right middle frontal gyrus, and bilateral central temporal gyrus. Puncturing right Heart 5 results in activation of the bilateral language related areas.

Heart 7, activates brain regions that are not identical, but both activate language implicated brain regions. "The coactivated Brodmann areas were Brodmann areas 22, 40, 44, and 47. Brodmann area 22 is one of the classical Wernicke's areas involving language understanding.

Pericardium 6

Pericardium 6 is located 2 cun above the wrist crease. PC 6 is a major point to regulate the stomach, and heart. It treats hiccups, by relaxing the diaphragm. It improves circulation in the chest to treat heart issues, and difficulty breathing. It treats the inability to speak, or loss of memory after a stroke. It also treats palpitations, where you feel your heart beating, nausea, insomnia, angina, and it strengthens the heart.

Make sure to not bend back your hand when locating this point. You can bend back the hand to locate the wrist crease, but move it back in a flat position for the correct measurement. If your hand is bent back, it will make the location off by quite a bit. I like to put vaccaria ear seeds on this point, but you can also just press firmly for five minutes. Treat the healthy side, to treat in this case.

Clenched Jaw

There is a chapter on jaw issues, but I wanted to include an image for the jaw points in this chapter also, in case you need it. Because these muscles are needed to speak. The points are Stomach 4, 5 ,6, and 7, and are explained in the lockjaw chapter.

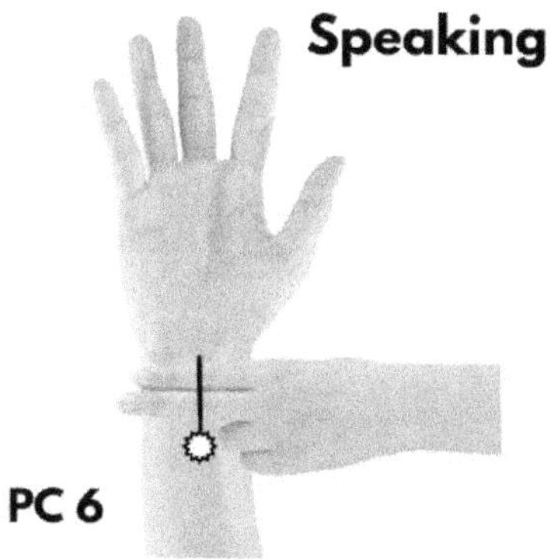

Points of last Resort - Points under Tongue

There are points inside the mouth, under the tongue, which are used to restore speech. I have not personally used these, but they are used in stroke clinics in China. I am including these points in case you need them, but I personally believe that any of the points in this chapter will work for you. As you might imagine, stimulating these points strongly encourages the restoration of healthy tongue function.

Acupuncturist Notes

Notes for acupuncturists who choose to treat these points. Ask patient to open mouth and stretch out tongue. Press on root of the tongue with depressor to expose base of the tongue. Insert needle perpendicularly 1 cun along base of the tongue. Maintain the needle below and parallel to the tongue body rather than inserting into the tongue. Or prick to bleed with a three-edged needle. Drawing more than 5 ml blood will give better results. There are videos online on how to treat these points.

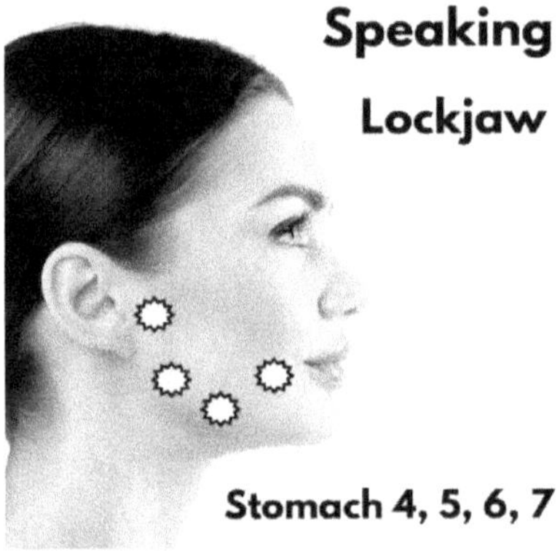

Speaking and Swallowing

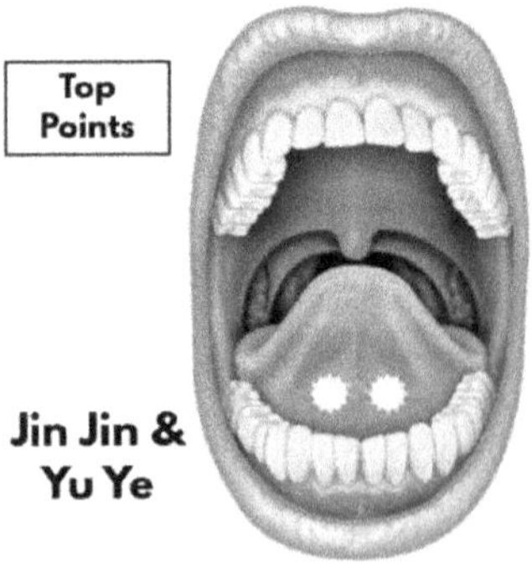

SWALLOWING

Swallowing difficulty or dysphagia occurs in 27 to 64% of stroke patients.

One of the dangers right after a stroke is that you might not be able to swallow. If your ability to swallow has been affected, you won't be able to drink or eat until that has recovered. Your medical team will test you and determine if it is safe for you to swallow. If you try to drink before you have been cleared to do this, it is possible to get food or drink inside your lungs, and choke.

After you are allowed to treat yourself with acupressure, you can press gently, but firmly on the points, and massage gently for about 5 minutes. If you are able to get vaccaria or ear seeds, or a mini massager, you can use that also. Be gentle in this area.

The ability to swallow depends on a lot of muscles. There are from 25 to 30 muscles that have to be functioning normally to be able to swallow safely.

In order to chew and swallow, you must make saliva. If your salivary glands have been affected by the stroke, they need to be treated also. Fortunately, there are acupuncture points that can help.

The esophagus, which is the tube from the mouth to the stomach, must be able to propel the food and liquid down to your stomach. This covers a large area. The stomach must also be functioning, because once the food arrives, it needs to process it, and send it on.

As you will see, swallowing is complicated. Since every stroke is different, you will need to determine which problems you have, and treat all of them.

This is an image of all areas that can affect the ability to swallow.

Swallowing and Digestion

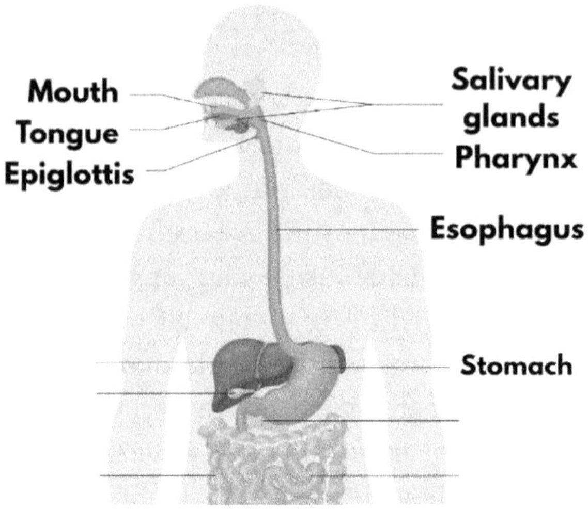

Small Intestine 17 is located between the angle of the mandible, which is the jawbone, and the anterior border of the sternocleidomastoid muscle. Just find the corner of your jaw bone, and beneath that on the neck is the muscle. Small Intestine 17 benefits the throat. It moistens the throat, to relieve difficulty swallowing.

Notice how some of the points used to treat swallowing problems, Triple Warmer 17, and Small Intestine 17, are located on or near salivary glands. They would not only relax the muscles in the face that restrict function, but they would improve salivation. They restore nerve function of the salivary glands.

Triple Warmer 17 is located behind the earlobe, between the jaw bone and mastoid process. It treats lockjaw, deafness, tinnitus, and dimness of vision.

Swallowing, Salivation

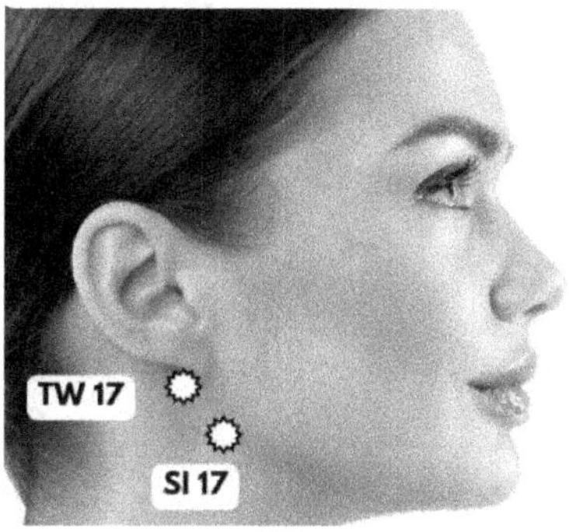

Swallowing, Salivary Glands

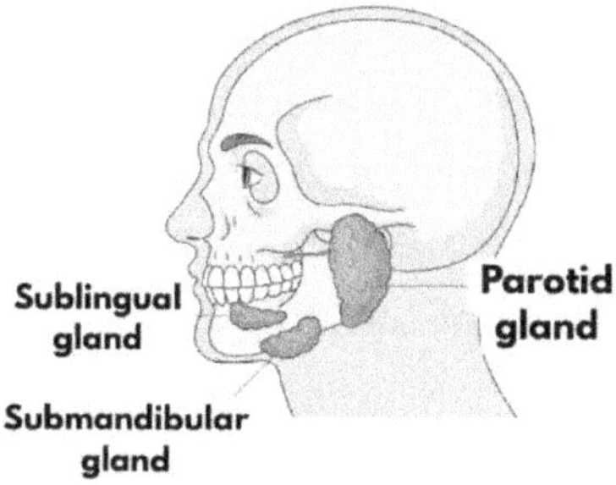

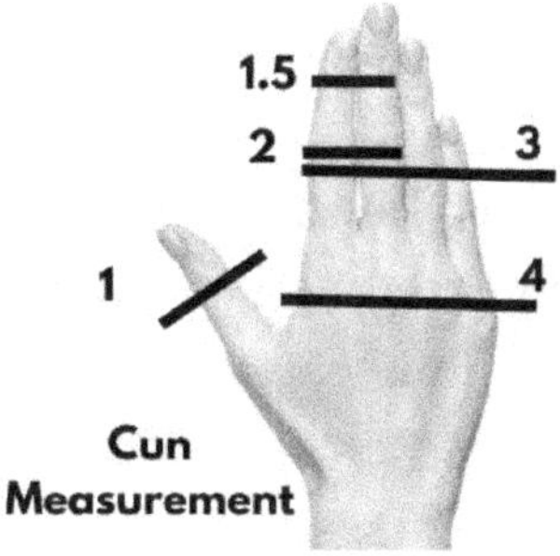

To treat swallowing problems, the most important points are Gallbladder 20 and Ren 23 on the neck.

Stomach and Esophagus

To treat the stomach and esophagus, activate Ren 12, and then treat the points above it. Ren 13, 14, and 17. Press firmly, into the muscle, and massage firmly. It is hard to miss the points if you just stay on a straight line above the navel.

Ren 12 is located 4 cun above the navel, on the midline. Use your hand to measure this, using the biggest knuckles by the hand, not the finger knuckles. Ren 12 is amazing to regulate your digestive system. It treats acid reflux, hiccups, vomiting, and it stimulates the stomach to send energy downward, instead of it flowing back up towards the throat.

Ren 13 is located 5 cun above the navel, on the midline. It regulates the stomach, and heart. It treats acid reflux, and nausea.

Ren 14 is located 6 cun above the navel, on the midline. It benefits the diaphragm, opens the chest, and regulates the heart and stomach.

Ren 17 is located at the level of the nipples, in the fourth intercostal space.

Ren 22 is located at the center of the suprasternal fossa. That is the hollow at the lowest point of your throat, above the sternum bone. This point moistens the throat. If lack of saliva is part of the problem, this point should help.

Ren 23 is located above the Adam's apple, in the depression of the upper border of the hyoid bone. It benefits the tongue. Due to the location of this point, it is not used much by acupuncturists. It is a tender area, and I would prefer acupressure on this point.

Swallowing

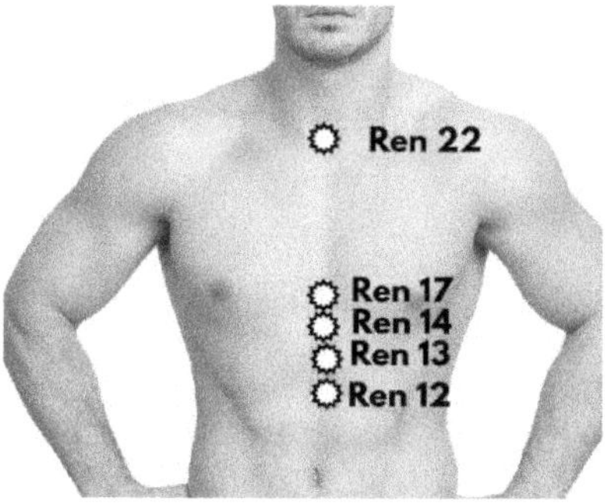

Some of the points to treat swallowing, also help speaking.

As you can see from this image, you can treat under the jaw bone, and down the throat. You will probably not need all these points. I would press firmly with the tip of your finger. I think a mini massager could be helpful for this, but check with your therapist and doctor. Remember that you can use the tip of the Sonicare toothbrush to activate this point, with the cap removed. Be very gentle. See what you can tolerate.

Ren 24 is located between the chin and the lips. Ren 24 relaxes the tendons in the face, treats deviation of the mouth and eye, lockjaw, facial paralysis, and neck pain. This point also helps to restore swallowing because it is located on the Ren meridian, which is on the midline, and affects everything on that meridian.

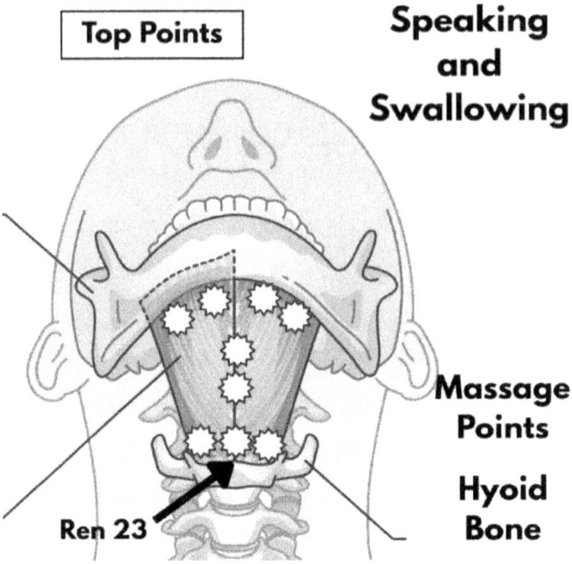

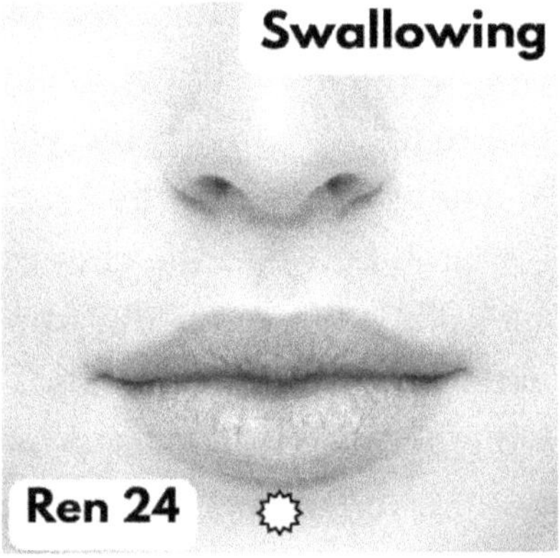

Gallbladder 12 is located in the depression behind, and below the mastoid process. This point can be difficult to find. Just feel the bottom of your skull behind your ear. Press in that area. A lot of muscles attach in this area, and you will probably not feel sure you have found it. Don't worry. There is no downside to massaging and pressing in the area in several locations to make sure you treated it.

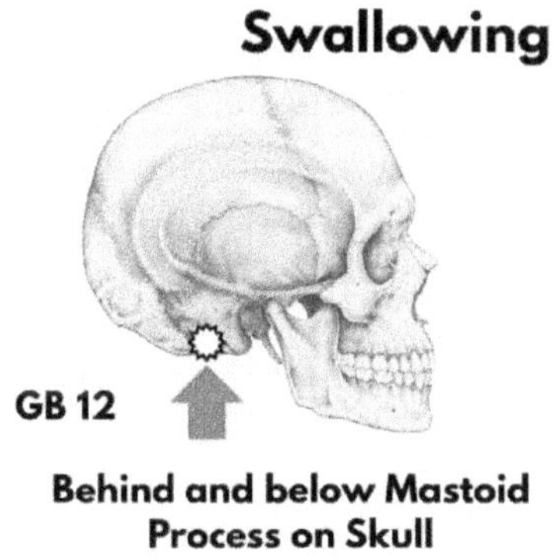

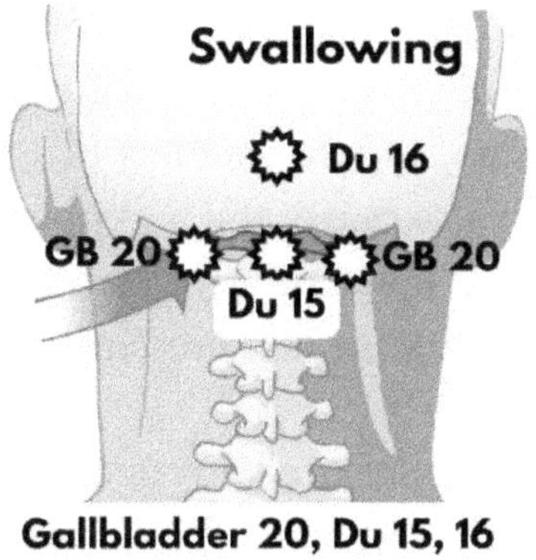

Gallbladder 20 is located in the hollow between the sternocleidomastoid and trapezius muscles, at the base of the skull.

Secondary Points on the Back of the Head

I believe that the points described above will be enough to restore the ability to swallow. But there are many other points that you can try, if you still need help. Please be sure to press firmly for about 5 minutes on each point, and treat daily with acupressure.

Du 15 is located one half cun above the posterior hairline, below the first cervical vertebrae. It is located opposite the root of the tongue. It benefits the tongue, and is used to treat the inability to speak after a stroke, tongue stiffness, and neck pain.

Du 16 is located 1 cun above the posterior hairline, in the depression below the EOP, or external occipital protuberance. This sounds complicated, but it is just the lump on the back of your skull. Du 16 treats difficulty swallowing.

Pericardium 6 is located 2 cun above the wrist crease, between the tendons of the forearm. Measure with your forefinger and middle finger, at the knuckles.

Pericardium 6 regulates the heart and stomach, it relaxes the diaphragm, which would help with hiccups, and breathing also. It treats nausea, and the inability to speak or loss of memory after a stroke. It is also one of the best points to treat insomnia. A Vaccaria seed would make the stimulation stronger on this spot, but I get great results with just pressing firmly. Press very firmly for 3-5 minutes.

Stomach 36 is one of strongest points on the body to regulate the digestive system. It is located 3 cun, which is one hand width, below the eye of the knee, by the shin bone. In my point location book, *Acupuncture Points Handbook*, there are three pages of information one what this point can do, but for this book, I will just include information on swallowing. Stomach 36 treats diaphragm spasms, difficulty swallowing, fatigue, hiccups, and indigestion.

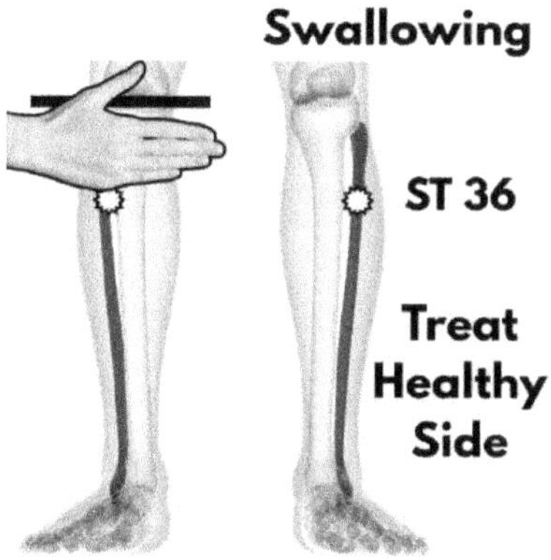

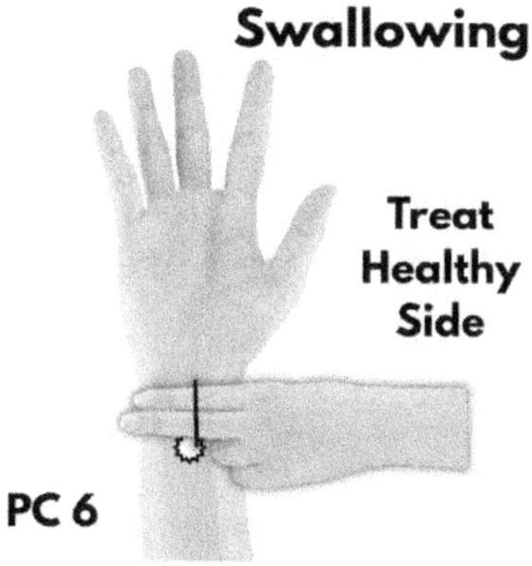

Secondary Points

There are points under the tongue, called Jin Jin, and Yu Ye, which are typically not used by most acupuncturists. They are specific to the tongue function. I would personally treat all the other points first, but if that is not enough, I wanted you to know about these points.

In China, some acupuncturists do bloodletting on these points. The goal is to get a drop, which stimulates the point. I have not personally treated these points, and would try all other points numerous times. But if you need another option, I wanted to make sure you have it.

When choosing acupuncture points, you usually have several options. So if someone doesn't like a point for some reason, there is an alternate point that also works. Licensed Acupuncturists will be able to be flexible on which points are chosen.

Notes for Licensed Acupuncturists Only

Ask the patient to open the mouth and stretch out the tongue, press the root of the tongue with a depressor to expose the base of the tongue. Insert the needle perpendicularly 1 cun along the base of the tongue. Maintain the needle below and parallel to the tongue body rather than inserting into the tongue. Note that the points are not on the tongue, but beneath it. If you want to use bloodletting, use a three edged needle and draw more than 5 ml blood for the best results.

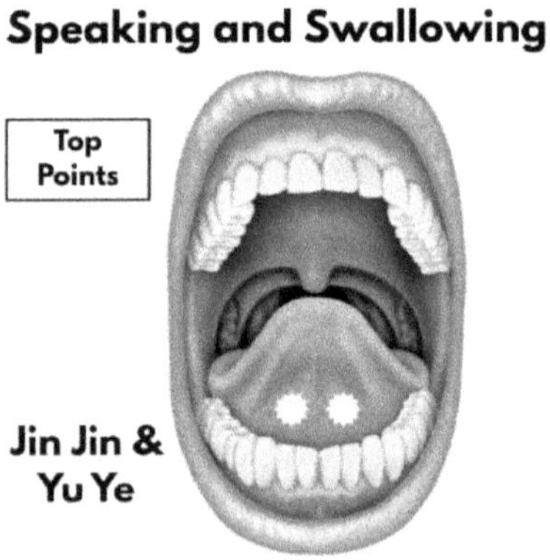

Swallowing Points on the Back

A few other options will be hard for you to locate, unless you are used to counting vertebrae. Acupuncturists do this all the time, but most people don't. We locate points on the spine by counting down the vertebrae. So, I suggest that you just press in the general area. There is no downside to massaging the area, so don't worry if you don't get the exact spot. Relaxing these muscles will make everything work better.

Bladder 16 is located 1.5 cun lateral to the spine, at the level of thoracic vertebra 6. It restores circulation in the chest, treats pericarditis, and diaphragm spasms.

Bladder 17 is located 1.5 cun lateral to the spine, at the level of thoracic vertebra 7. Bladder 17 regulates the diaphragm to treat hiatal hernia, esophageal constriction, and acid reflux.

Bladder 46 is located 3 cun lateral to the spine, at the level of thoracic vertebra 7. It regulates the diaphragm. It treats belching, hiccup, and vomiting.

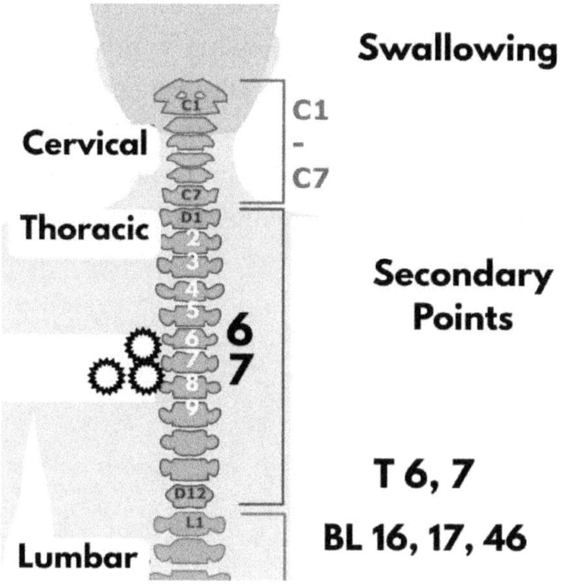

Modern Explanation of Swallowing Acupuncture Points

The anatomy of these points is Gallbladder 20 is located in the sensory fiber innervation areas of the glossopharyngeal, hypoglossal, and vagus nerves, with the vertebral artery and medulla oblongata in the deep layer. A study showed that stimulating this acupuncture point could improve blood supply to the cerebral artery.

Ren 23 is at the root of the tongue. Sensory afferent fibers in the hypoglossal nerve and glossopharyngeal nerve can be found in these areas, and the glossopharyngeal muscle group is dominated by the submaxillary hyoid muscle, the anterior abdomen of the digastric muscle, the genioglossus muscle, the pharyngeal constrictor muscle, and the cricothyroid muscle.

These nerves and muscles represent the structural basis for normal swallowing function. An existing study revealed that conducting acupuncture at the above acupoints could directly stimulate nerve terminal receptors and reflexively enhance the regulation ability of the swallowing center in the brainstem. Accordingly, efferent impulses are transmitted to the effector muscle to realize the reconstruction of the swallowing nerve pathway and the recovery of neuromuscular function.

Dysphagia is typically considered to be worse for liquids than solids.

VISION

When stimulating any points around the eyes, please do not use a mini massager. This is too strong for the eye area. Simply pressing for five minutes should be enough. Vaccaria ear seeds can be placed on the points for stronger stimulation. Make sure to consult your physical therapist or doctor for this. You might be unable to sense the location very well after a stroke.

About 20 to 60% of stroke patients have vision problems. Patients might not even know they have a problem with their eyes until they have an eye test. My mom had problems with her peripheral vision, but she was not aware of it, until she was evaluated by her eye doctor.

Having a problem with peripheral vision could make it more dangerous to drive. If you don't know you have an eye problem, you could easily miscalculate distances. If you can, get an eye test as soon as you can after a stroke, to determine what issues you might have.

Even if you are not sure about the state of vision, you could gently treat the eyes with acupressure. The points used for the eyes are standard points that improve vision. You can ask your doctor about this. Make sure you use a mirror if you treat yourself. The points are easily activated and the area around the eyes is very sensitive. There are about 50 points on the body that are known to benefit the eyes, but these points are the first choice.

There are muscles on the outside of the eyeball, which move the eyeball around. Just as the muscles and nerves in the rest of the body do not function normally after a stroke, any muscle on the outside, or the muscles around the optic nerve can be affected.

Eye movement problems can be caused by the nerves which control the muscles around the eyes. In the same way that your arm does not move as well, your eye muscles can be affected also. This affects eye focus, and muscle movement.

Vision problems can include visual processing problems which cause you to struggle to understand visual information. You might not notice or recognize things located on the affected side of your body.

You do not have to know what is causing your eye problem. Acupuncture points work to regulate and restore healthy function.

The type of visual problem is determined by the area of the brain that is affected by the stroke. It is not necessary to know which area was affected, the acupuncture points work on the whole area. You will need to be evaluated by your eye doctor, but some potential eye problems include:

- Light sensitivity
- Dry eyes
- Gaze palsies cause the inability to move both eyes together in the same direction
- Eye movement disorders
- Droopy eyelids
- Reduced visual sharpness
- Visual field defects cause reduced ability to see when looking left or right, this makes it dangerous to drive
- Ocular dysmotility, the eyes do not align
- Blurred vision
- Smooth pursuit disorder affects the ability to follow moving objects
- Saccades, which is reduced fast eye movement
- Visual neglect is when a portion of the visual field is affected
- Anisocoria – when one pupil is bigger than the other

- Nystagmus is a vision condition which causes the eyes to make repetitive, uncontrolled movements. These movements often result in reduced vision and depth perception and can affect balance and coordination. These involuntary eye movements can occur from side to side, up and down, or in a circular pattern.

Vision Points

Bladder 2 is one of the most important points to treat vision, and it is located at the inner end of the eyebrow. This point is often used instead of Bladder 1, which is at the inner canthus, which is very close to the eyeball. Bladder 2 opens and brightens the eyes. It can be used to treat glaucoma, optic nerve atrophy, color blindness, blurred vision, and sudden blindness.

Gallbladder 1 is located .5 cun lateral to the outer canthus of the eye, on the bone. Gallbladder 1 brightens the eyes, which means it restores healthy circulation in the eyes. It treats glaucoma, night blindness, optic nerve atrophy, and Lasik Dry Eye. Just press firmly on the bone. The eye area is very sensitive, and be very careful where you are pressing. I used Gallbladder 1 to quickly restore normal tear production after I had Lasik Eye Surgery. It stimulates the lacrimal gland, which is the gland that produces tears.

Yu Yao is translated as Fish Waist. It is at the midpoint of the eyebrow. It benefits the eyes. It treats eye pain, and drooping eyelids. This point improves circulation in the eye, and it treats the muscle that lifts the eyelid. It is located directly above the pupil of the eye when looking directly ahead. The arch of the eyebrows is not a reliable locator. Use the pupil.

Stomach 2 is located directly below the pupil, on the lower border of the eyeball socket. This is not in the eye orbit, but below the eye orbit bone. It treats excess tear production, trigeminal neuralgia, nearsightedness, color blindness, and eye pain.

Tai Yang is translated as Supreme Yang. The description of its location sounds very complicated. It is about 1 cun, or thumb width, behind the midpoint between the lateral end of the eyebrow and the outer canthus. That probably makes no sense at all. It is used to treat eye disorders, vision problems, eye pain, and deviation of the mouth and eye. Remember that the points are an area, not a pinpoint, so just do your best.

Du 17 is called “Brain’s Door”. It clears the brain, and benefits the eyes. It can be used to treat blurred vision, and tinnitus. As a side note, it corresponds to the visual cortex area of the brain. It is located 1.5 cun above the EOP, which stands for external occipital protuberance. It is a bony ridge or knot on the back of your skull. I bet you always wondered what that knot was.

Gallbladder 20 is located at the base of the skull. Press on this point, and the area around it, for five minutes on both sides of the head. It is often sensitive in this area, because a lot of muscles attach there, and they can be tight.

Gallbladder 20 is a very important point that is used for about 100 things. It treats blurred vision by improving circulation to the eyes, treats loss of speech after a stroke, and it also opens blocked ears, among many other things.

Do Not Use any Massager by Your Eyes or Ears

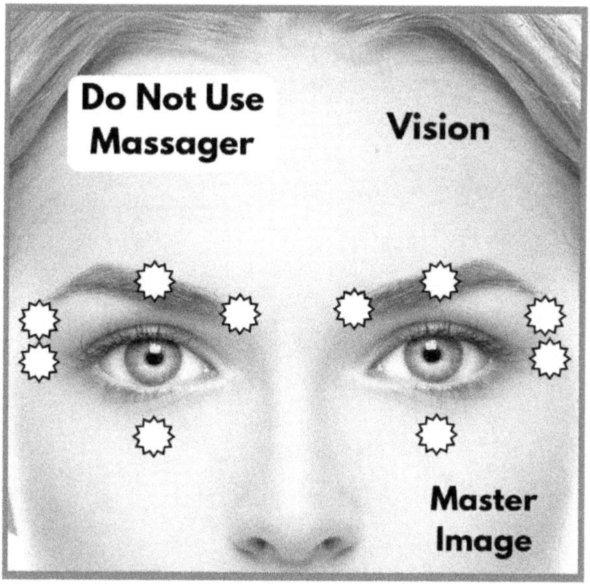
Do Not Use
Massager
Vision
Master
Image

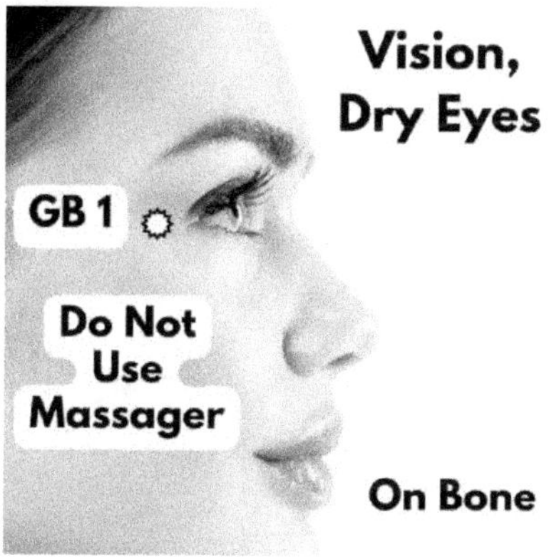
Vision,
Dry Eyes
GB 1
Do Not
Use
Massager
On Bone

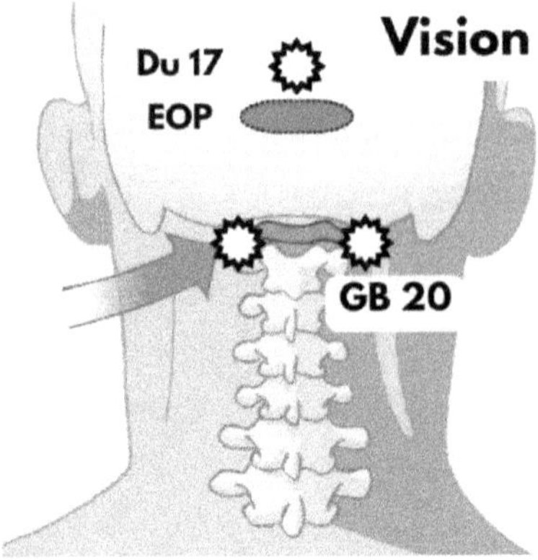
Vision
Du 17
EOP
GB 20

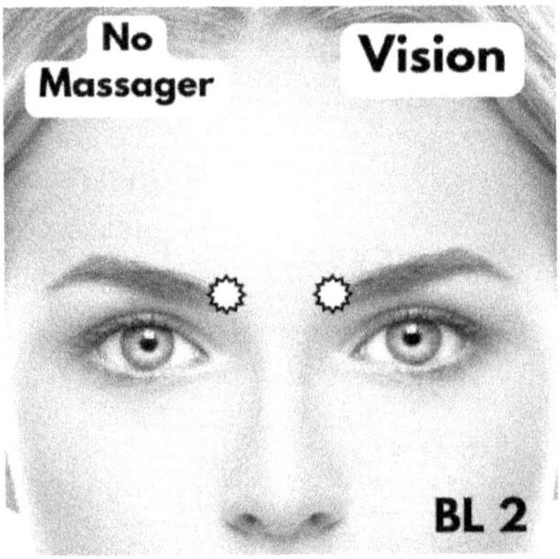
No
Massager
Vision
BL 2

Vision

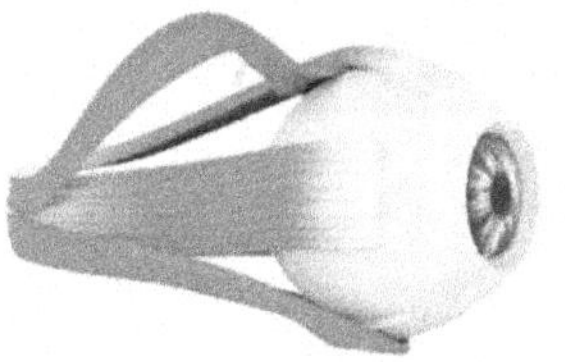

Eye Muscles

Vision

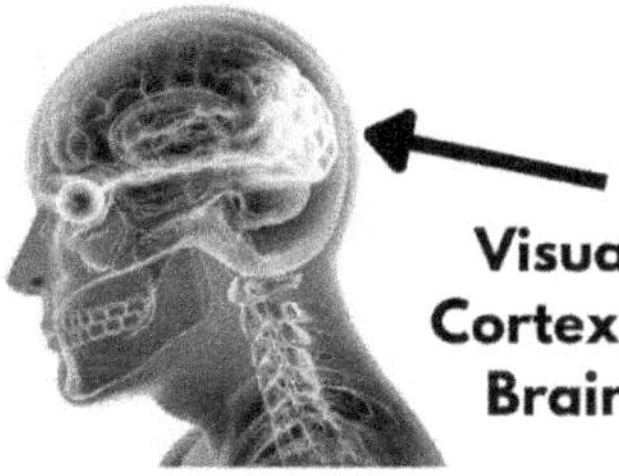

Visual Cortex of Brain

Vision, Dry Eyes

Tear Gland

GB 1

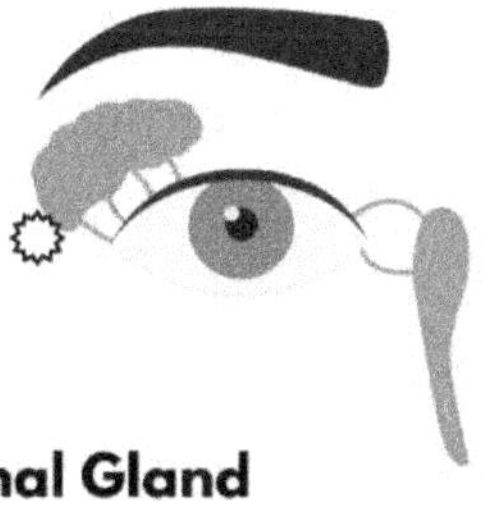

Lacrimal Gland

CHAPTER 5

CHEST, TRUNK, ABDOMEN, AND DIGESTION

Bladder Incontinence

This chapter explains how to treat bladder incontinence, the inability to urinate, all urinary problems, and weak-stream urination. Activating the points in this section regulate the bladder, and restore function.

Bladder incontinence affects about 40% to 79% of stroke patients. This can improve on its own, but 25% to 33% still have bladder issues when released from the hospital or treatment center. One year after a stroke, 10% to 15% of patients still have bladder incontinence.

Chinese medicine excels at treating all bladder issues. It is very easy to treat this, and most people have no idea how effective Chinese herbs are to treat incontinence, or bladder weakness of any kind.

The most important acupuncture points to treat bladder issues after a stroke are located on the midline, just below the belly button. I would treat all the points starting one inch below the belly button, all the way down to the pubic bone. Stimulating these points helps to restore function in the bladder.

Press firmly for about five minutes per point. If you had bladder issues before your stroke, you might need to treat more times to resolve the issue. I will also explain some herbal remedies which can help.

Ren 2 is located directly below the navel, on the upper border of the pubic symphysis bone. It treats the inability to urinate, and incontinence. This point is not used a lot in clinic, due to its location above the pubic bone. Ren 3 is more commonly used, but in case the other points did not work, you have the option to use Ren 2.

Ren 3 is located 4 cun directly below the navel. This is measured by using the hand knuckles, the ones closest to the hand. Not the finger knuckles. Ren 3 treats bladder issues, regulates the uterus, and strengthens the kidneys. It is also helpful for bladder pain.

Ren 4 is located 3 cun directly below the navel. It treats fatigue, restores body energy after collapse, strengthens the kidneys, treats the bladder, and urinary incontinence. This is the most important point to treat.

Ren 5 is located 2 cun directly below the navel. It regulates the uterus, strengthens the kidneys, and treats difficult urination.

Ren 6 is located 1.5 cun directly below the navel. It treats kidney stones, rectal prolapse, uterine prolapse, and strengthens the kidneys.

You can see from the location of these points, on a line directly below the navel, that you can start at the top and treat one point after another. You don't need to worry about exact locations, because they are close together, and with acupressure, there will be overlap.

Incontinence after a stroke is treated differently than incontinence caused by other issues. Chinese medicine treats regular incontinence and weakness by strengthening the kidneys with Chinese herbal medicine. Most people need help with this as they age, as in Chinese medicine theory, the kidneys weaken over time, and need to be strengthened.

If you have a catheter, you are more likely to get an infection. Bladder infections can kill you. The bacteria can easily spread from your bladder to your kidneys and cause a kidney infection. It can also cause sepsis, which is deadly. If you have any symptoms of a bladder infection, make sure to get it tested, if you have any suspicion at all.

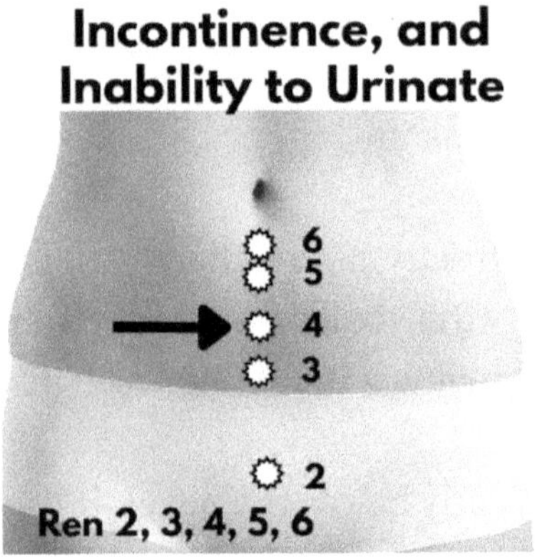

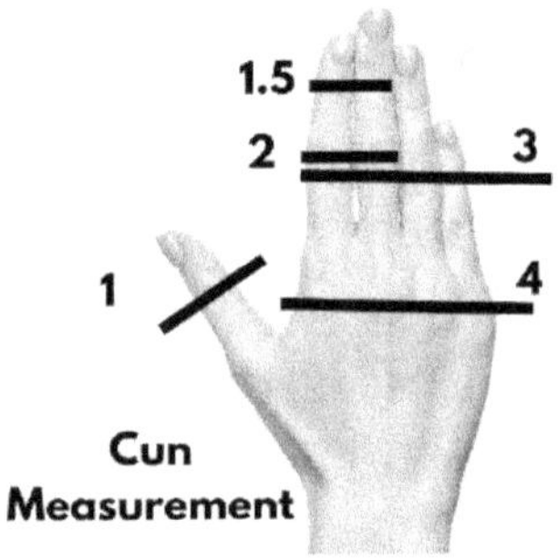

Common symptoms of a bladder infection include a strong urge to urinate, burning sensation when urinating, passing frequent and small amounts of urine. Your urine could be cloudy, or dark. You might also have pain in your bladder area.

Kidney infections can escalate to sepsis if the infection spreads to the bloodstream. Sepsis is a major cause of death, with over 270,000 deaths annually in the U.S.

As an acupuncturist, I use Chinese herbal formulas to treat bladder infections. In Chinese medicine, it is seen as heat in the bladder. The herbs clear heat. I don't want you to substitute this for antibiotics from your doctor, but I want you to know there are natural options.

One of the formulas Licensed Acupuncturists use is called Chuan Xin Lian, or Antiphlogistic. It has been used to treat bacterial infections for centuries. The most common formula is Andrographis, dandelion root, and Isatis root. Kan Herbs Antiphlogistic is a good option.

If one of my patients had a suspected bladder infection, I always refer him or her to a medical doctor, but prescribe the herbal formula Chuan Xin Lian. You can keep this formula in your medicine cabinet to get started on killing bacteria, before you can see your doctor. Oregano oil, and olive leaf extract might also be helpful.

Some people take cranberry juice, thinking it will treat a bladder infection. It is not strong enough. It does not kill bacteria. It reduces the adherence of bacteria to the wall of the bladder, but that is not enough. A bladder infection should always be treated urgently.

If you had weak bladder symptoms before the stroke, that usually means you have weak kidney energy in Chinese medicine. Most bladder weakness problems can be resolved within a month with the right Chinese herbs.

There are many kidney tonic herbs in Chinese medicine, but I would not recommend taking them without a prescription, because there can be side effects. These herbs can increase testosterone, which can cause excess facial hair in women. This problem usually goes away once the herbs are no longer taken.

An over-the-counter herb that can help is cordyceps. This is a fungus and it is used in Chinese medicine to strengthen the lungs, kidneys and heart. I recommend only the fruiting body extract, and the brand I prefer is Freshcap Mushrooms. I usually suggest two pills, twice a day. It strongly boosts energy levels.

Make sure to ask your doctor about any supplements before you take them.

To treat weak bladder and incontinence, you can also do acupressure on Kidney 3 and 7, by the inner ankle bone. These points strengthen the kidneys and are the first choice. Press on the points for 5 minutes on both legs.

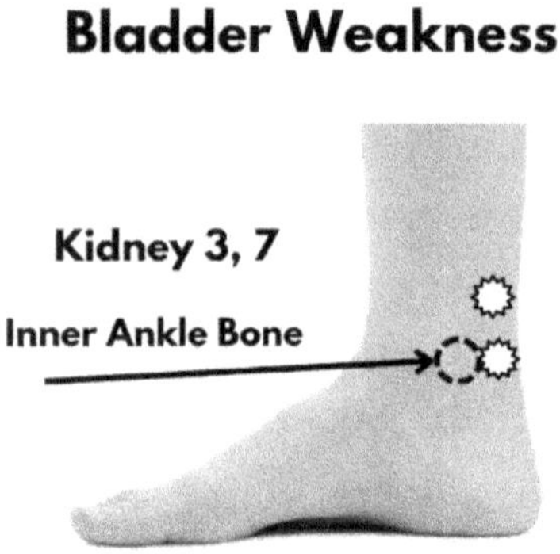

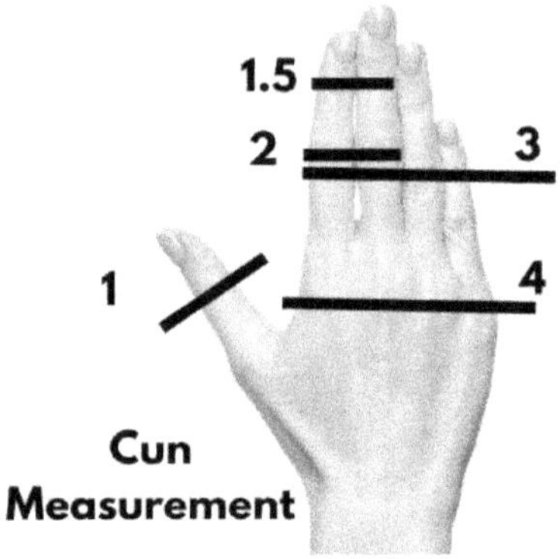

Constipation

Constipation is very common after a stroke. It affects between 29 and 79% of patients. Many people were already constipated before they had a stroke, so this needs to be treated. Sitting in bed after a stroke, and being in a care facility can make it more likely to be constipated.

It is important to have a bowel movement at least once a day. Probiotics are very helpful to treat constipation. Most of the stool is bacteria, and if you don't have enough bacteria, you will not have a healthy stool. I like Primal Defense from Garden of Life.

A good laxative is ground flax seeds. You can sprinkle them on your food, or put a tablespoon in hot water and drink. The liquid is enough of a laxative, but you can eat the flax seed also. Be sure to clear this with your doctor or nurse. What concerns me about taking a laxative is that if the nerves in the colon are not working, it could cause problems. Ask your doctor or nurse for permission to take any supplement.

There are several points on the abdomen that regulate the colon. Press and rub very firmly, until you feel an achy sensation, and maintain it for five minutes.

Stomach 25 is located 2 cun lateral to navel or midline. It treats abdominal pain, constipation, diarrhea, intestinal abscess, intestinal obstruction. It moistens and regulates the intestines to treat constipation, and diarrhea.

Stomach 27 is located 2 cun below navel, 2 cun lateral to the midline. It treats abdominal distension. It strengthens the kidneys to improve urination, and treat painful, and difficult urination.

Stomach 28 is located 3 cun below navel, 2 cun lateral to midline. It treats retention of urine and stool, painful urination, abdominal distension, genital pain, and constipation.

Spleen 15 – Located at the level of the navel, 4 cun lateral to the midline. It treats constipation, fecal incontinence, and regulates the intestines.

Large Intestine 11 – Located halfway between the elbow crease and the elbow. Locate with the arm slightly bent. This point is number one to treat constipation. Press very firmly for 5 minutes, with your thumb on your healthy hand. I would treat both arms. The healthy arm will probably act faster to regulate the colon, but treating the affected arm will improve arm function, and activate colon function.

Large Intestine 11 moistens and moves the intestines. You can easily grab this point with your thumb. It can also be used in the bathroom, if you are sitting there and not getting results. Keep pressing until it works. It is one of the most dependable acupressure points, with obvious results.

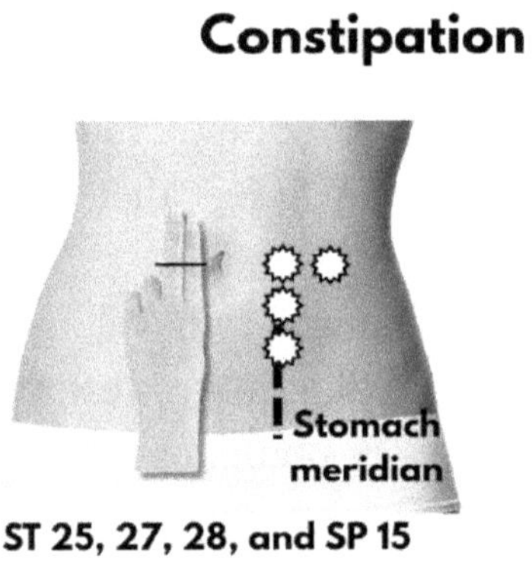

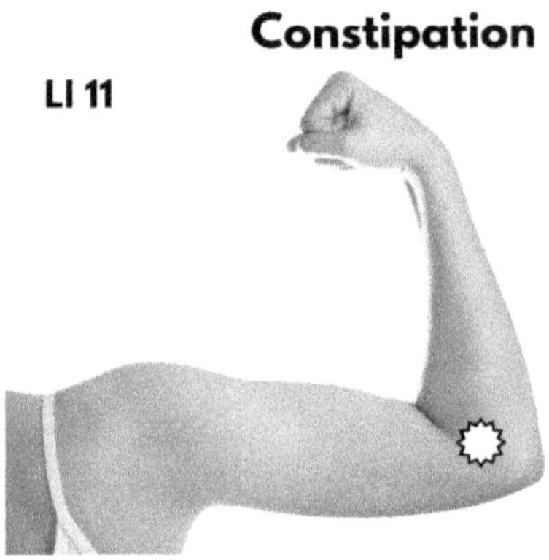

Diarrhea

Diarrhea can be caused by many things. It might be caused by the stroke, affecting the nerves in your colon, but it could also be caused by eating food you are not used to, or the stress of being in a care facility. It affects 30% to 40% of stroke patients.

Fecal incontinence is when you cannot control your stool, in the same way urinary incontinence is the inability to control your bladder.

Ginger root is my favorite herb to treat diarrhea. You can take three capsules of ginger root, or put it in hot water and drink it as a tea. You can also take probiotics like Primal Defense by Garden of Life to restore the good bacteria in your colon.

The points in this section regulate the function of the colon. Notice these are the same points that treat constipation. They regulate the intestines, treating whatever imbalance you have.

Spleen 15 – Located at the level of the navel, 4 cun lateral to the midline. It treats constipation, fecal incontinence, and it regulates the intestines.

Stomach 25 -Located at the level of the belly button, 2 finger widths away. This point is a major point to treat digestive disorders. It treats abdominal pain, colitis, constipation, diarrhea, edema, intestinal obstruction, pancreatitis, and vomiting. It regulates the intestines, that is why it treats both diarrhea and constipation.

Just start at the level of the belly button, two fingers away, and work your way down, pressing firmly for about five minutes.

Stomach 36 and 37 are secondary points. You will probably not need them. I would focus on the abdomen first. Stomach 37 is located 3 cun below stomach 36, one finger width lateral from tibia bone, the shin bone. Stomach 37 treats diarrhea, gastritis, indigestion, intestinal obstruction, leg pain and numbness, leg weakness and atrophy. It regulates the intestines and stomach, and resolves stagnation in the intestines.

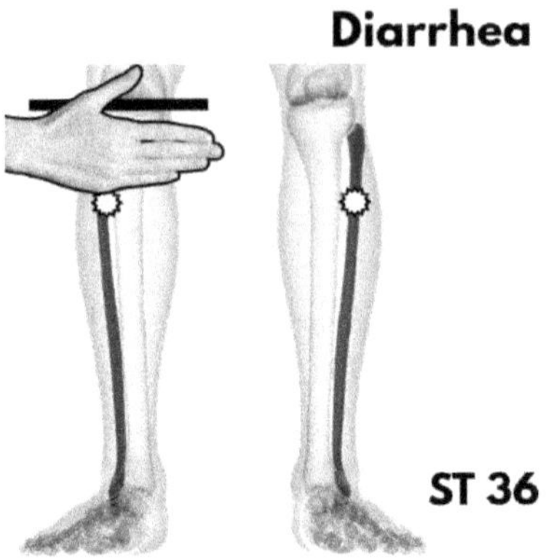

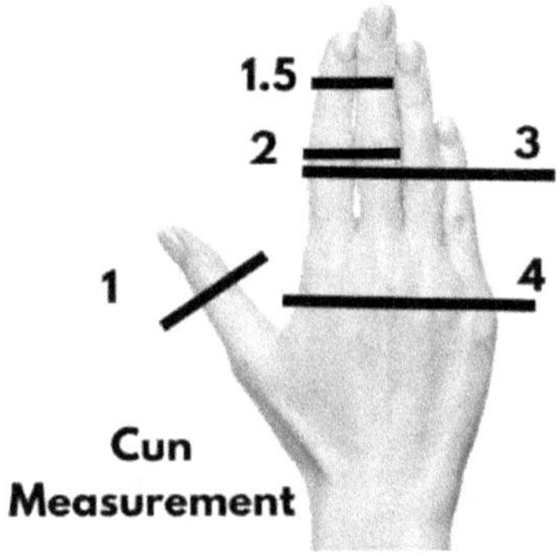

Diarrhea, Fecal Incontinence

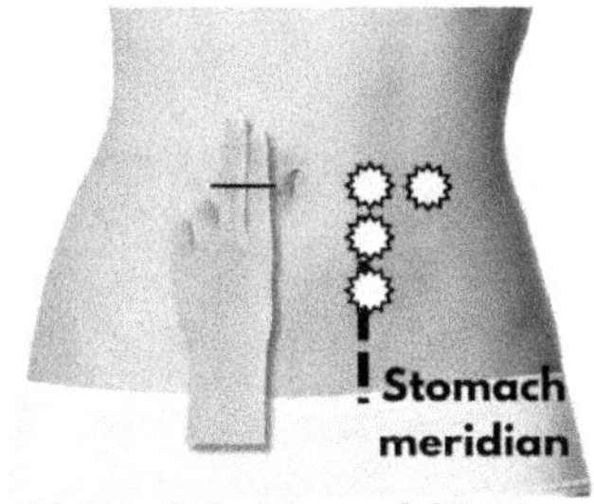

ST 25, 27, 28, and SP 15

Treat Healthy Side

Diarrhea

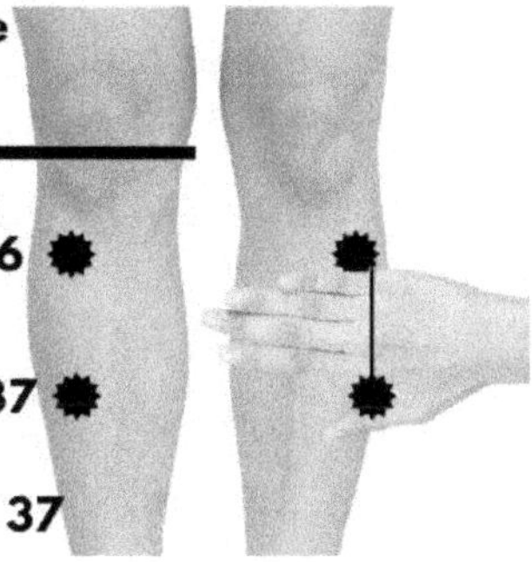

CHAPTER 6

SHOULDERS, ARMS, AND HANDS

This chapter includes the whole arm, starting from the shoulder, down to the fingers.

After a stroke, the shoulder muscles can be weak, or suffer from spasticity. If the muscle function is not restored, the upper arm bone can slip out of the joint, which is called a subluxation, or partial dislocation. The muscles have to be strong enough to hold the arm bone in place.

Over time, the muscles that are not used can become stiff, or the range of motion of the shoulder can be affected. Keep moving your arm as much as possible, or the muscles can tighten up and it can take months to loosen them up again. Your physical therapist will give you exercises to restore your arm function. Do them. If you don't, your arm problem will get worse over time.

Applying heat to the shoulder can help to relax the muscles. You can use a heating pad, hot water bottle, or a ThermaCare heat patch, and apply to the areas where you feel the most pain, that is often where the muscles are too tight. Relaxing the tight muscles is very important to treat this.

Shoulder Hand Syndrome

Shoulder Hand Syndrome is pain in the arm which is caused by a stroke. Restricting blood flow to any area will starve the area of oxygen and nutrients. It cannot heal. If this goes on too long, the nerves and muscles develop other problems.

You might have swelling, extreme nerve sensitivity, skin changes, or further reduction in the ability to move the arm. In Chinese medicine theory, all pain is caused by stagnation. Stagnation is a blockage of blood flow. When the blood flow is restored the pain goes away, because the tissue now has enough oxygen and nutrients to function normally.

Cold Shoulder or Arm

If your arm or shoulder is cold, you need to warm it up. If it stays cold, that means the circulation is not good. It will be hard for the body to heal if the blood flow is impaired.

After my dad's stroke, his leg was cold. I applied heat to it repeatedly, and it warmed back up. I also did acupuncture on his calf muscle, and massaged his leg as heat was applied. It took about two hours to warm his leg up. I had a limited amount of time to treat him, so I just kept working on his cold leg. It would not have warmed up on its own, and it might have been a long-lasting impairment. I believe that if I had not applied heat, he would not have healed as well as he did.

Whatever you do, do not apply cold packs. Applying cold, even if you think the inflammation will be reduced, will not help. Inflammation is your body's way of healing itself. Applying ice will further restrict circulation. It has been proven that the body will actually compensate for the application of cold by increasing inflammation later. Some people will disagree with that. Gentle heat is all you need.

Arm Spasticity

Spasticity is when the muscles cramp up. You can lose control over your arm. It is caused by a failure to resolve the lack of circulation in the arm. Spasticity can occur any time after a stroke. It takes time for your brain to heal, and symptoms can pop up out of nowhere until it is fully healed.

Shoulder Points

Large Intestine 15 is located in the front part of the shoulder joint. It is used to treat shoulder and arm pain. When treating arm pain, or hand problems, it is common to treat Large Intestine 15, 11, and 4. Treating these points on the meridian is a strong way to activate circulation in the shoulder, arm, and hand. These are your most important points.

The images that say Master on them include numerous points in one image, to make it easier for you to treat them. I then break down the points separately to explain them.

Press and massage very firmly on each point for five minutes. If you can get a mini massager that will help. Remember that you can use your Sonicare toothbrush, with the cap removed, to activate the points also. Just use the tip of the brush. It is actually pretty strong.

You just need a massager that is small enough to focus attention on a smaller area. Treat twice a day as soon as you can after your stroke. Don't give up. You should see benefits after a few treatments, but if your stroke was not recent, it might take longer.

Deltoid Muscle Lifts the Arm

The primary muscle responsible for lifting the arm is the deltoid muscle. Notice that many of the acupuncture points are located where the muscle attaches.

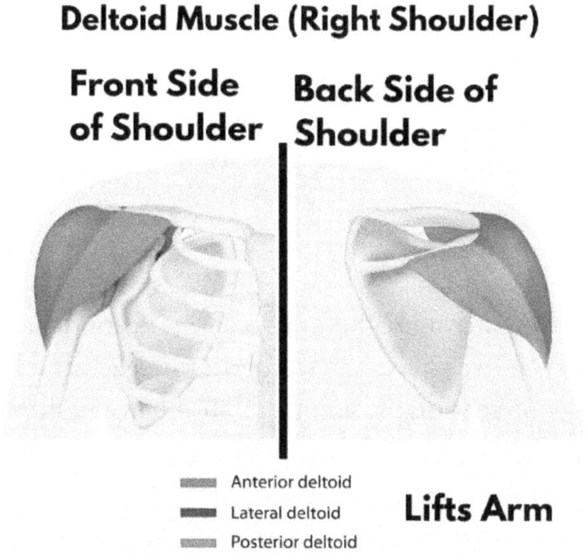

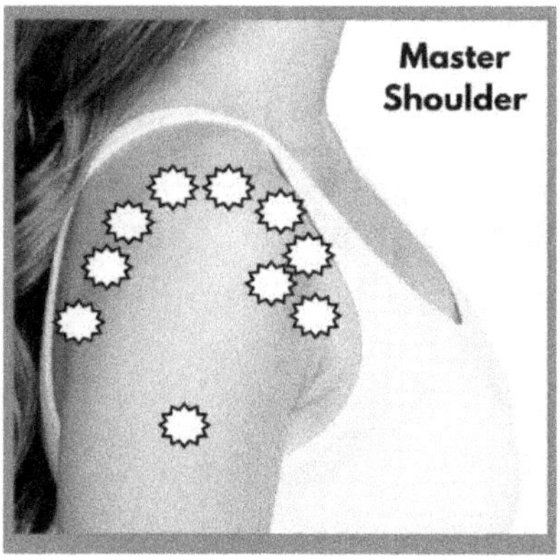

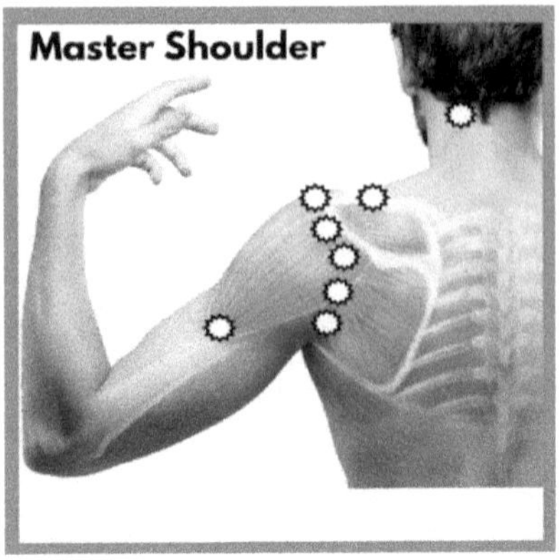

Be sure to surround the entire shoulder on the front and back. The image above shows the shoulder muscles attached to the shoulder blade, or scapula. If you treat all the areas shown with a star, and you still cannot lift your arm, treat it again. In order to use your arm at all, you need to be able to lift it.

It will take a little time to activate all the points on the front and back of the shoulder. If you need to rest, that's OK. Be patient with yourself.

After you treat the shoulder, you will want to move your way down the arm. The Large Intestine points to treat are starting at the front of the shoulder, Large Intestine 15, moving down by the elbow, to Large Intestine 11, and 10, then to Large Intestine 4. These are the most important points on the arm to restore arm function.

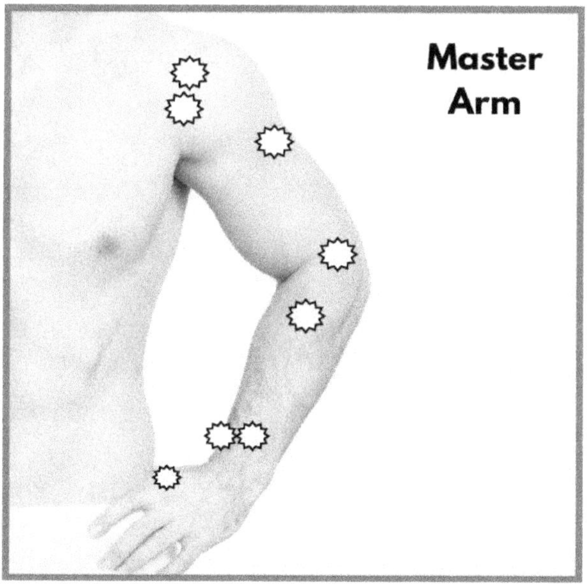

However, just treating the Large Intestine meridian is not enough. It might help you lift your arm again, but it will not restore the muscles that move the forearm and hand. If you do not treat those also, you will not be able to write as well, and you might get problems with your hand or fingers, where they go into a spasm, and cause a claw hand.

In Chinese medicine theory, muscle spasms are caused by a lack of blood supply. When the blood flow is blocked, the muscles become starved of oxygen, and other nutrients, and go into a spasm to pull blood into the muscles. Doing acupuncture, acupressure, or massaging the acupuncture points will restore blood flow, stimulate the nerves to send signals to the brain and restore function. Heat also increases blood flow.

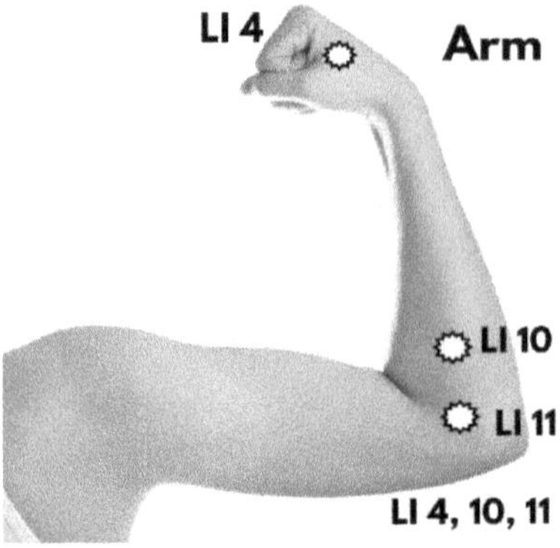
LI 4
Arm
LI 10
LI 11
LI 4, 10, 11

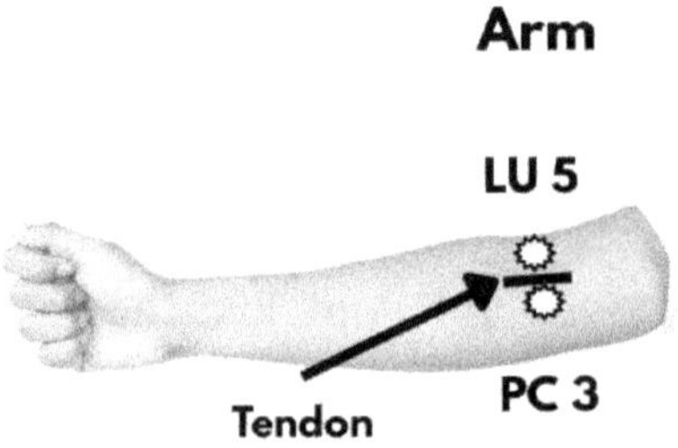
Arm
LU 5
Tendon
PC 3

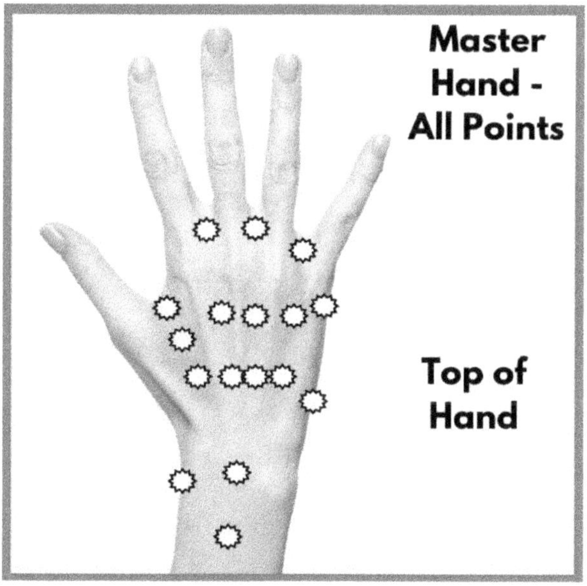

Finger Contraction

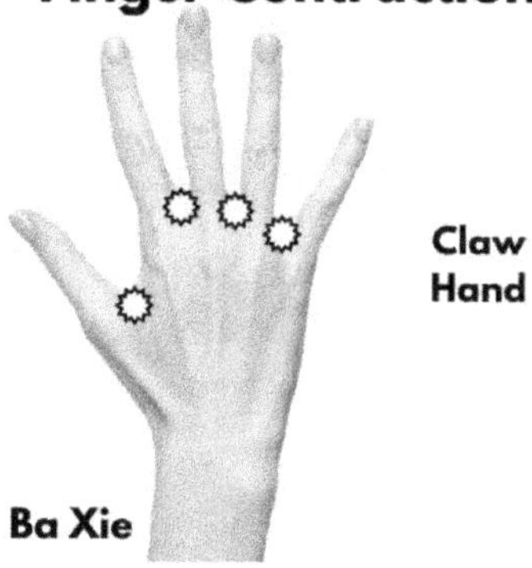

Be sure to treat the hand, forearm, upper arm, and shoulder, because you won't know which areas have been affected in isolation. Just treat them all.

Small Intestine 3 is located at the knuckle by the little finger. This is a major point. It treats elbow pain, finger pain, hand pain, headache or neck pain, stiff neck, and many other things. It is also used to restore circulation in the hand and Small Intestine meridian.

Small Intestine 4 is located at the base of the fifth hand bone, and the triquetral bone. This is the round bone of the wrist. It treats wrist contracture and stiffness, finger pain, and hand weakness.

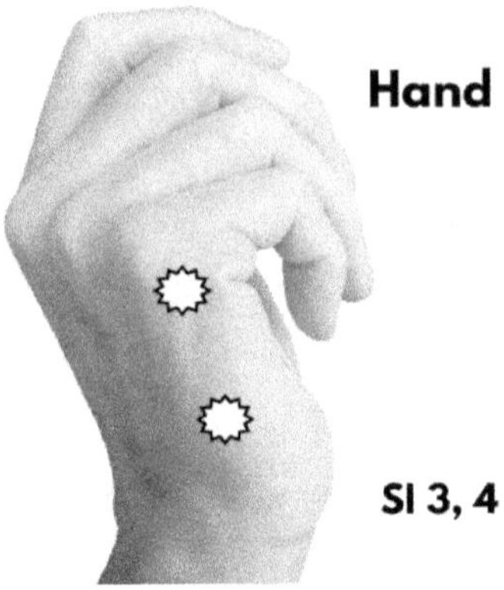

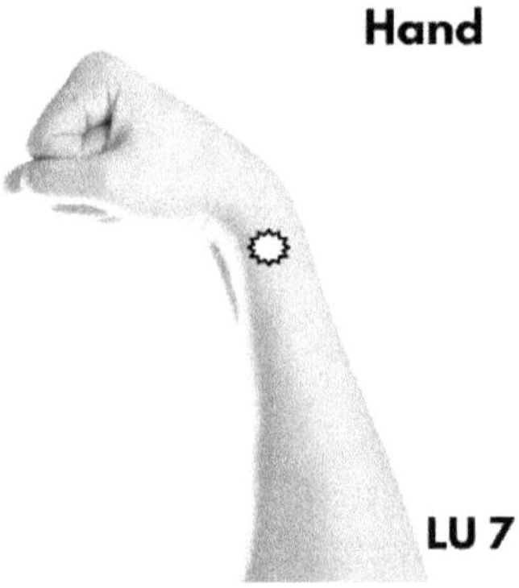

Hand

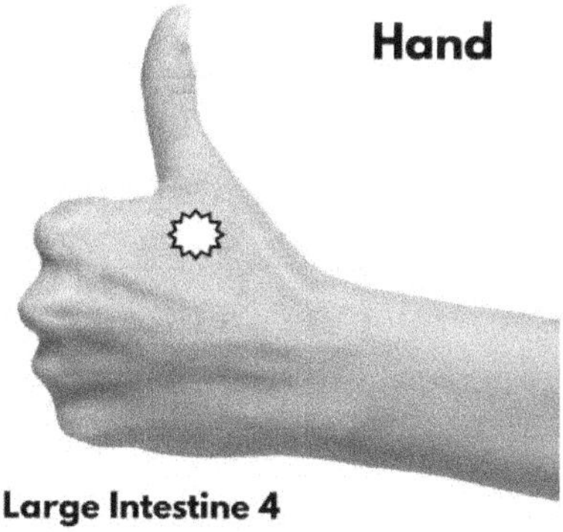

Large Intestine 4

Hand, Forearm

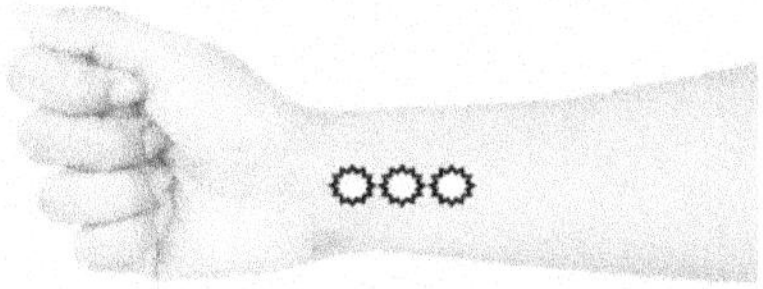

Pericardium 5, 6, 7

Large Intestine 4 is located between the first, and second hand bones. Find the fleshy area, not the skin. It will be tender. This point treats hand pain, allergies, headaches, hives, and many other things.

Pericardium 5 is located 3 cun above the wrist crease, between the tendons. This point treats the Heart, and Pericardium energy. It is also listed as treating drooling caused by a stroke. Although I would also treat the muscles around the mouth.

Pericardium 6 is located 2 cun above the wrist crease, between the tendons. This is a major point with dozens of uses. The top functions are treats anxiety, stomach issues, heart arrhythmia, and it also restores healthy circulation in the chest. It also treats the inability to speak, or loss of memory after a stroke. It is popular to treat nausea due to any cause. In this case it is used to restore circulation in the hand and arm.

Pericardium 7 is located in the middle of the wrist crease, between the tendons. It regulates the heart to treat insomnia, and it also regulates the stomach. Treating these three points together will improve circulation in the hand and lower arm.

Ba Xie, also called Eight Pathogens, are located between the fingers. These points treat numbness, stiffness, and pain in the fingers and hand. These points can be used to treat any nerve, or pain problem in the hand, and arm. They strongly stimulate the restoration of circulation in the hand and arm. To treat these points, spread the fingers of the affected hand, and use a mini massager. You could also try Vaccaria, or ear seeds.

Spasticity or Contraction of Arm or Hand, Claw Hand

Ask yourself what causes claw hand, spasticity, or contracture of any muscle? In the case of a stroke, the muscle is not getting an adequate signal from the brain, to ensure a healthy blood supply.

You just need to treat the affected areas, so blood flow and healthy nerve function are restored. If you want to understand how this works, use your healthy hand and make the same position that your affected hand is in.

In order to make your hand go into a claw shape, you will have to use your forearm muscles, as well as your hand muscles. You can feel and see the muscles in your arm move, when you put the hand in the claw hand position.

If you are able to get acupuncture or acupressure soon after your stroke, I believe that you will be less likely to have contractures or spasticity. In the event you do have this problem, there are specific points that are especially helpful to treat that.

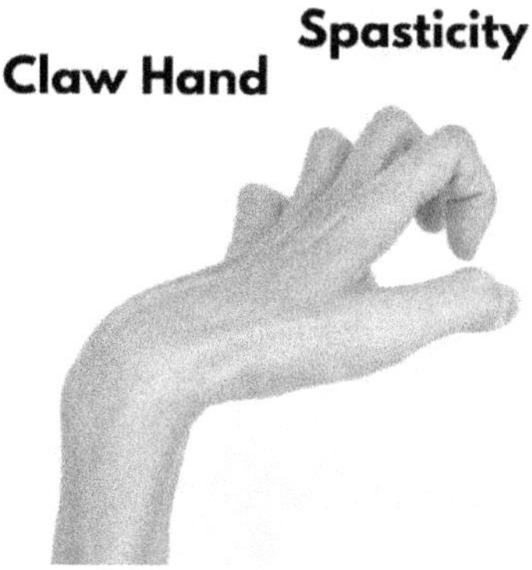

Keep Your Muscles Warm

You could use an electric blanket or throw, and keep the muscles warm. After a stroke your circulation might be impaired, so you will want to add heat therapy to relax the muscles and speed healing. Be careful to not overheat, because your ability to sense heat levels might be reduced.

Shoulder Subluxation

A shoulder subluxation is when the humerus, or upper arm bone, slips out of shoulder joint. This is also common with broken arms. The points to use include TW 14, Jian Nei Ling, LI 14.

As long as your shoulder and arm muscles are weak, or not used enough, the bone will be unlikely to go back into the joint. A subluxation will not likely resolve on its own. If you no longer have the help of a physical therapist, there are many videos on YouTube showing you exercises you can do.

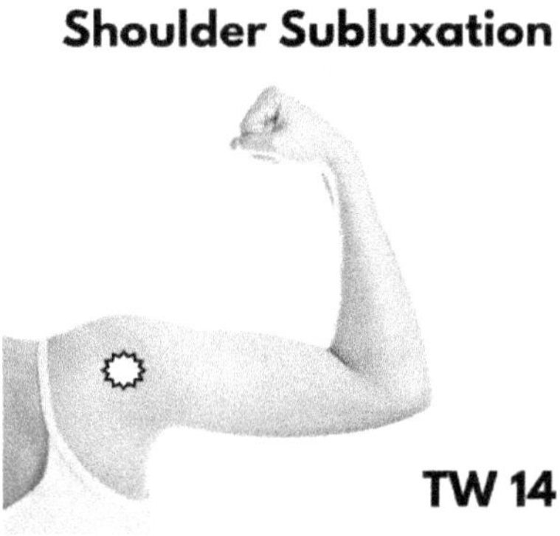

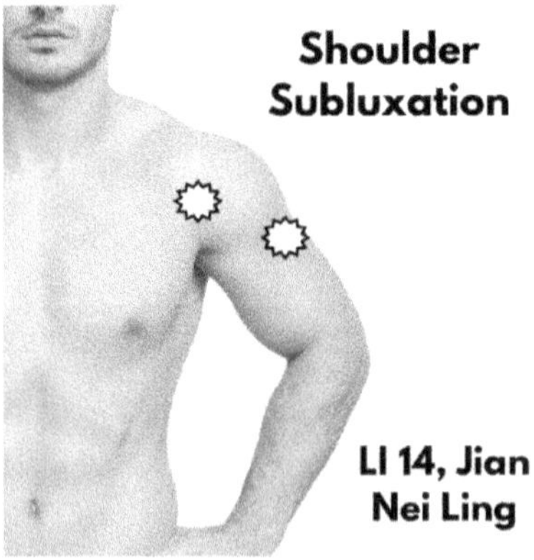

Shoulder Subluxation

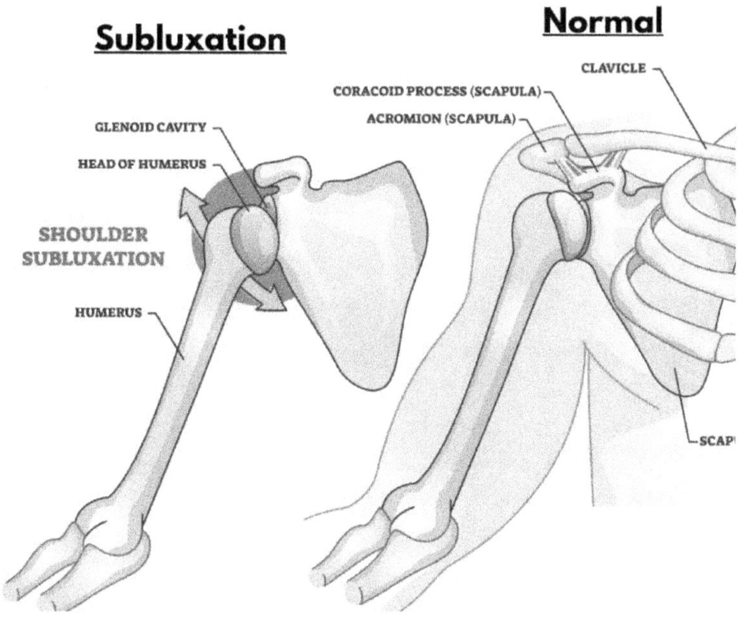

Wrist Contraction

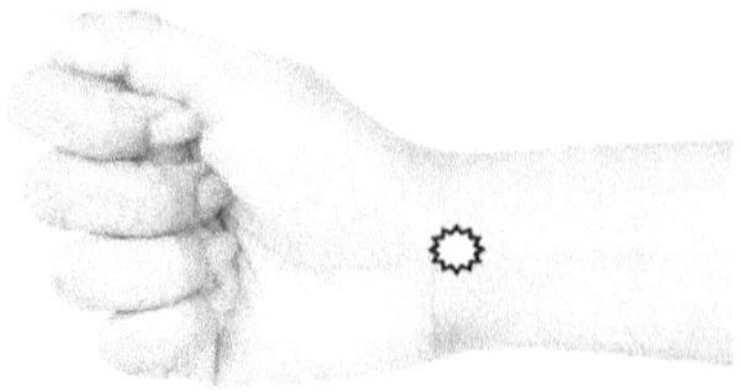

Pericardium 7

Elbow Contraction

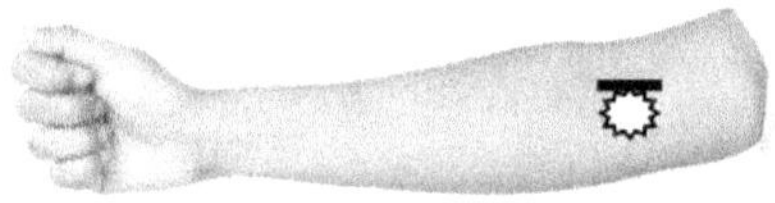

Pericardium 3

Handwriting Extra Points

In addition to the points already listed for the hand, and arm, treating these points, which are not listed acupuncture points, will treat the smaller muscles that will help you write well again. LI 4 on the top of the hand will do a lot of what you need to treat the thumb, but I believe treating the palm side of the thumb is very important.

There is currently no acupuncture book, or scientific reference, that includes all the acupuncture points that stroke patients need. So I have done research on which muscles perform specific functions, that are affected by a stroke. The points in the handwriting section are in addition to regular acupuncture points.

In order to be able to write, you need to be able to hold the pen with your thumb, as well as maneuver it with your hand muscles. These muscles might have been activated when you treated the hand points called Ba Xie, but to make sure you get them all, I would add additional areas on the hand and forearm.

Just use a mini massager for a few minutes per point. Press firmly, because there are several layers of muscles to reach. There is no way to know for sure exactly which muscle has been affected. So treat all of them.

You probably won't be able to get your massager between the bones in the hand, don't worry about that. Just do acupressure for a few minutes per point, and move on to next. Treating the palm side of the hand will most likely also treat the top side.

Handwriting

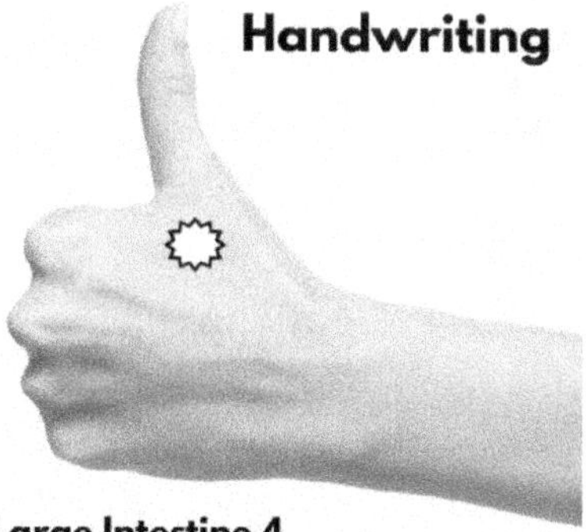

Large Intestine 4

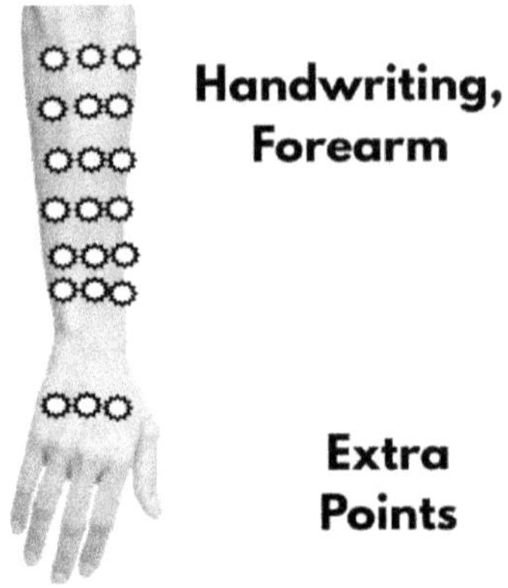
Handwriting,
Forearm
Extra
Points

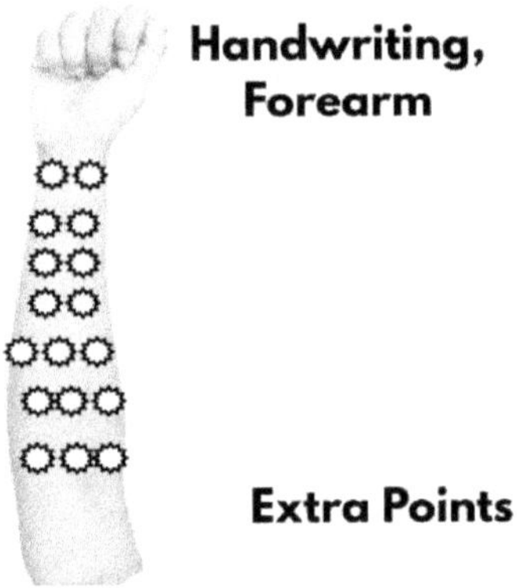
Handwriting,
Forearm
Extra Points

Handwriting, Palm

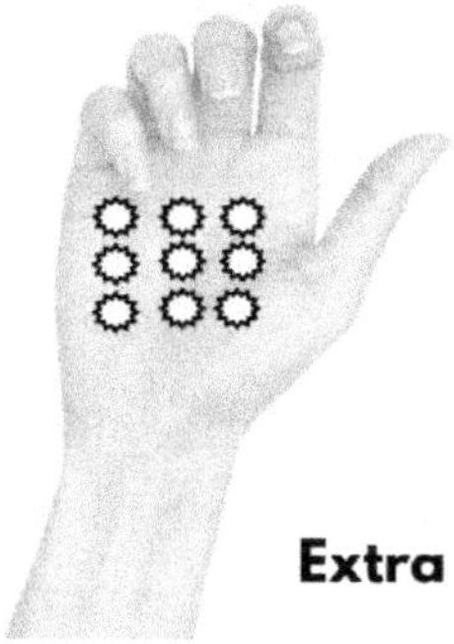

Extra Points

Handwriting, Thumb

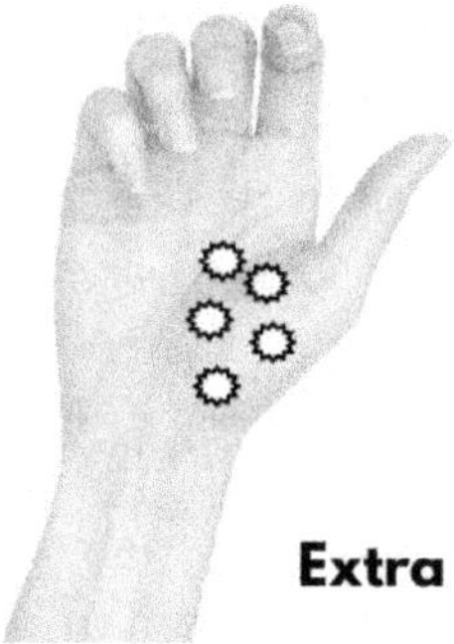

Extra Points

CHAPTER 7

HIPS, LEGS, FEET

This chapter includes the hip, knee, leg, and foot, including foot drop, and cold legs. It is difficult to break things out by area, because they are all connected. If you treat your feet, it benefits your whole leg. If you treat your knee, it benefits your whole leg. So, some sections run together.

To treat the area from the hip to the toes, I would start with the toes. The toes are on the end of the limb, and acupuncture points are particularly strong at the ends of limbs. If you are able to get results when treating the feet, working your way up to the knees, then the thigh, you might not need a hip treatment. Every person is different.

- Start on the foot and toes
- Treat calf muscles along shin bone, from knee to foot
- Treat calf muscles, front and back side

Treat the affected leg first. You can treat both legs at any time. If your problem is chronic, such as a month post stroke, treat both legs. Treating one leg also treats the other leg.

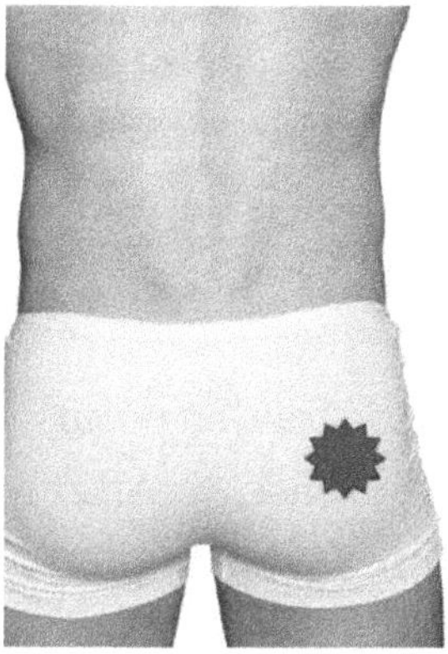
Hip
GB 30

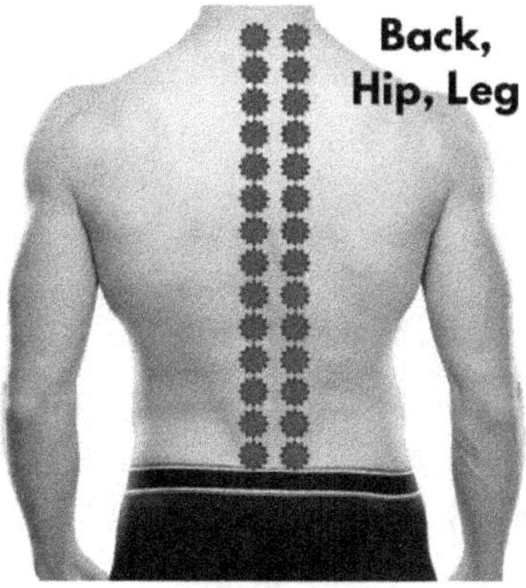
Back,
Hip, Leg

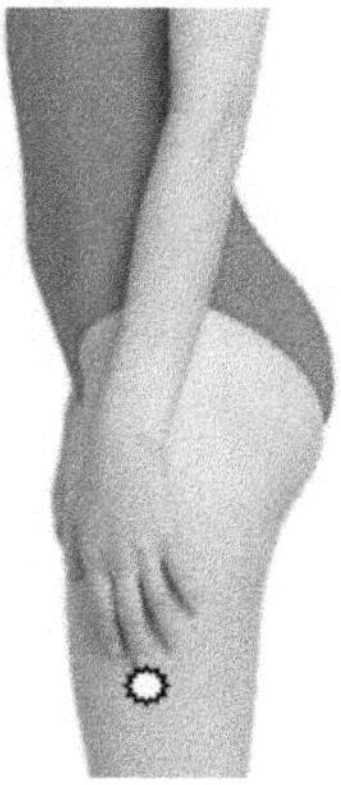
Leg
GB 31

Gallbladder 30 is a commonly used point to treat hip pain. It is also used for sciatica. It relaxes the hip muscles, and restores circulation in the area. The point location is described as one third of the way from the head of the thigh bone, and the top of the sacrum.

For hip pain, I treat the most tender points in the area. Points are usually tender due to tight muscles. After a stroke, you might be numb, or have no sensation. Just press very firmly to get to the muscle in the hip. Apply gentle heat before you do acupressure. You can relax with gentle heat for hours before treating.

Gallbladder 31 is located on the side of the thigh, where the tip of the middle finger touches the thigh. This point treats hemiplegia, knee and thigh pain, and leg weakness.

Knees to Toes

The following points are used to treat knee pain. They restore circulation in the knee joints, and the entire leg. I have used them to treat leg tremors. Pain, and the inability to use a limb is caused by a blockage in the meridians. Restore circulation in the strongest meridians, and that can often treat any type of problem in the leg, as these meridians affect the entire leg. You just use the key points on the meridian.

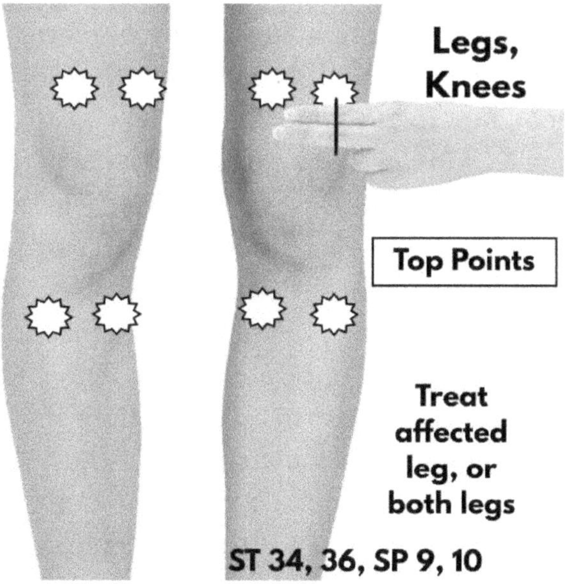

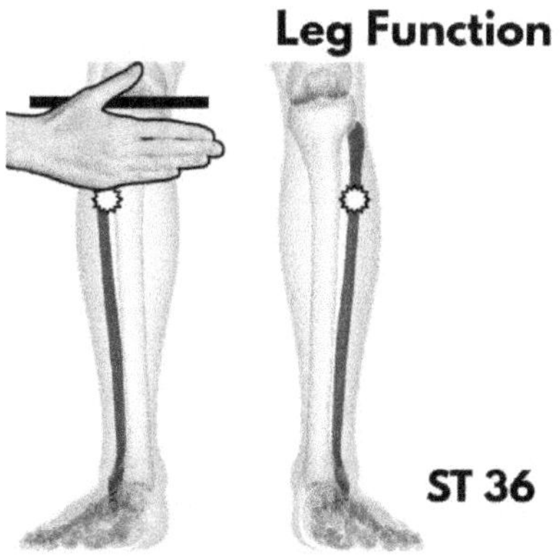

Spleen 9, 10, Stomach 34, 36 are used to treat knee pain. They restore healthy blood flow to the knees, so the pain is relieved. They also restore circulation in the leg, so I personally include them when treating leg, or foot neuropathy.

Spleen 9 is located in the depression by the knee, that is at the end of the tibia bone. It also treats edema, or fluid retention.

Spleen 10 is located 2 cun from the upper border of the kneecap. It treats knee pain, and regulates the blood. It helps to improve blood flow in the body.

Stomach 34 is located 2 cun above the upper border of the kneecap. It treats knee pain and swelling, and leg pain.

Stomach 36 is one of the most important points on the body. It is used to improve energy levels, treat digestive and immune issues, and anemia. It also treats leg pain, paralysis, and weakness. In my point location book, *Acupuncture Points Handbook*, it takes up 3 pages to list all the things Stomach 36 will do. It strongly improves circulation in the leg. There are two common ways to locate the point, you can measure down from the eye of the knee, using your hand, as shown in the image. You can also locate using the tibia, or lower leg bone.

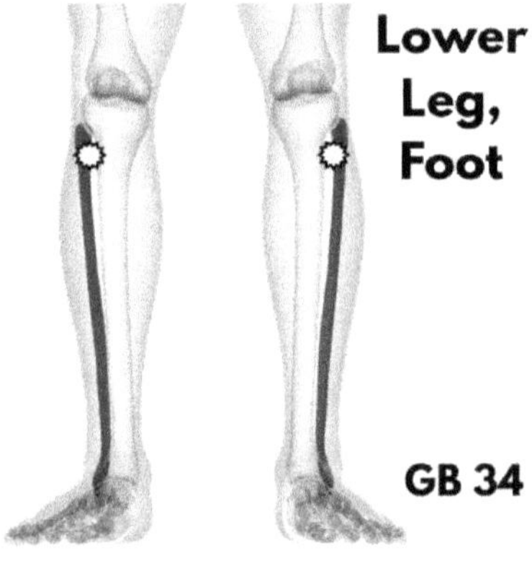

Gallbladder 34 is located at the depression in front of and below the head of the fibula bone. It is harder to locate than a lot of points. It is not far from Stomach 36. Just treat the area and points around it, to ensure you get the point.

Gallbladder 34 treats calf muscle atrophy, contraction of foot tendons, hemiplegia, and knee pain. It also relaxes the tendons to relieve muscle spasms. It can treat spasms anywhere in the body. It also can be used for nausea, and gallstones. For stroke recovery it also restores circulation in the leg.

When locating Gallbladder 34, start at the top of the fibula bone, which is the smaller bone on the outside of the calf, and move your way down to the lump you feel. There are wide variations in anatomy and the size of people's bones. Just treat the general area. Press and massage deeply for about five minutes, and treat the whole area. There is no downside to this. The more you do, the better. Don't worry that you are missing the point, because the points are an area, not a pin point location.

Front of Hip, Leg

Stomach 31 is located at the level of the pubic bone, on the upper thigh. Locate the pubic bone at the front of the body, and move toward the hip bone. Be careful to find and treat the muscle, not the fat. You could lie on your healthy side to get full access to this point. If you are lying down on your back, the fat, and muscle on your leg will spread out and make it harder to find. This is a tricky one to find, but it is worth it. Stomach 31 treats leg and hip atrophy, or paralysis. It also treats hip and leg pain, and numbness.

Front of Hip, Leg

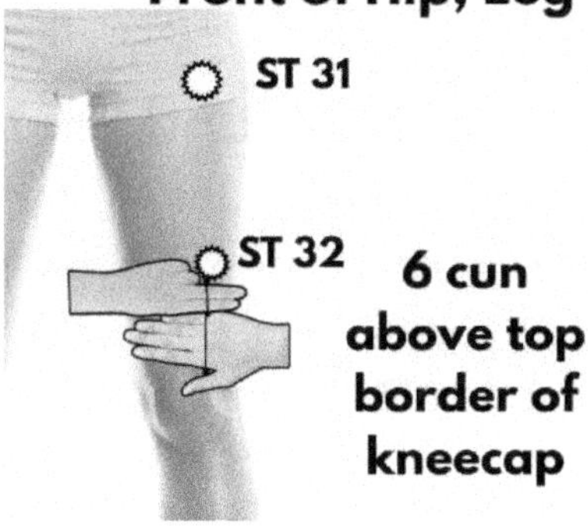

Stomach 32 is located 6 cun above the upper border of the kneecap. It treats knee pain, and paralysis of the knee muscles. Use one handwidth for 4 cun, and add two more. Press very firmly on this point, as it is located in a big muscle and needs strong stimulation to activate it.

Bladder 37 is located 6 cun below Bladder 36. I have included Bladder 36 in the image just to show you where it is located. Bladder 36 is in the gluteal fold, underneath the buttocks. You need only treat Bladder 37. Bladder 37 treats lower back pain, sciatica, and atrophy of the leg. Be sure to treat both sides of the leg and hip. This point restores circulation in the thigh.

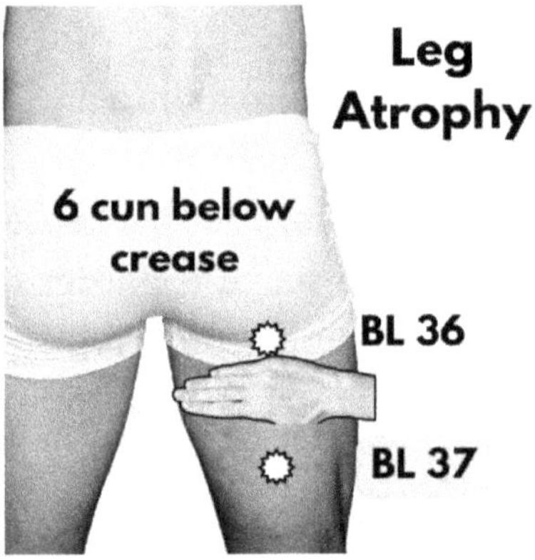

Lower Leg, Foot, and Foot Drop

The lower leg should be treated on the front, side, and back. The calf muscles must be working in order to lift the foot.

The following points are used to treat the feet. They are also used to treat foot drop. In treating foot drop, you need to treat the feet, and the calf muscles. It is also helpful to know which muscles lift the foot. All of these muscles, on the front and the back side, need to be treated.

The muscles that primarily lift the foot upward are the Tibialis Anterior, Extensor Digitorum Longus, Extensor Hallucis Longus, and Fibularis Tertius. The Tibialis Anterior is the main muscle that lifts the foot, while the other muscles assist in this action and also control the toes during the walking process.

Treating the muscles where they attach at the top of the leg, around Gallbladder 34, and Stomach 36, as well as where they attach near the ankle is a good idea. I would also treat the muscles themselves. You never know for sure exactly which muscles are affected, and where, so to prevent future problems I would start at the top of the muscle and spend 4-5 minutes per spot, and move my way down the leg to the foot.

Bladder 40 is located on the back of the leg, behind the knee. This point is famous to treat back pain. It will restore circulation in the leg.

Bladder 57 is located below the belly of the gastrocnemius muscle, on the back of the calf. It treats lower back pain, heel pain, and calf pain.

Foot Points, Foot Drop

Bladder 60, BL 60, is located between the outer ankle bone, and the outside of the ankle. It treats lower leg paralysis, lower leg pain, pain in the sole of the foot, heel pain, and lower back pain.

Bladder 61 is located directly below Bladder 60, in the depression of the heel bone. It treats foot atrophy, foot drop, heel pain, and lower back pain.

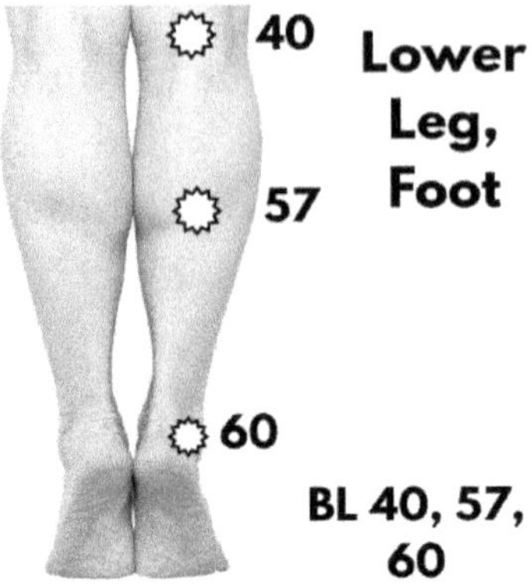
40
57
60
Lower Leg, Foot
BL 40, 57, 60

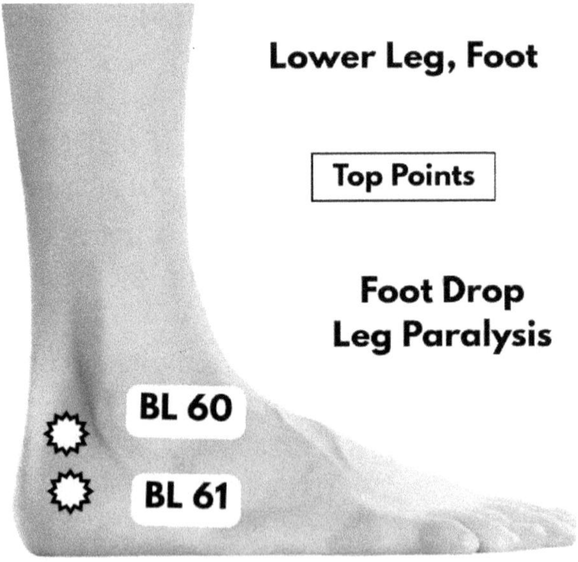
Lower Leg, Foot
Top Points
Foot Drop
Leg Paralysis
BL 60
BL 61

The points on the Gallbladder meridian will be a little harder to find. If the foot or leg is swollen, it will be even harder. Just find the outer ankle bone, and treat points around it. These points are important to treat foot drop, and leg atrophy. You might not need them, but they are here for you if you do.

Gallbladder 37 is 5 cun above the outer ankle bone, called the lateral malleolus, on the front of the fibula bone. It treats lower leg atrophy and pain, as well as it is a top point for vision problems. It treats eye pain, twitching, and blurred vision.

Gallbladder 38 is 4 cun above and in front of the outer ankle bone, on the front border of the fibula bone. The outer ankle bone is the end of the fibula bone. It treats tendons and bones.

Gallbladder 39 is 3 cun above the tip of the outer ankle bone, behind the fibula bone. It treats foot and leg weakness, and ankle sprain.

Gallbladder 40 is located in front of and below the outer ankle bone. It treats foot drop, and leg pain.

8 Winds is the English name for Ba Feng. These points are amazing to treat any nerve pain in the feet. They are located between the toes.

Toes, Foot

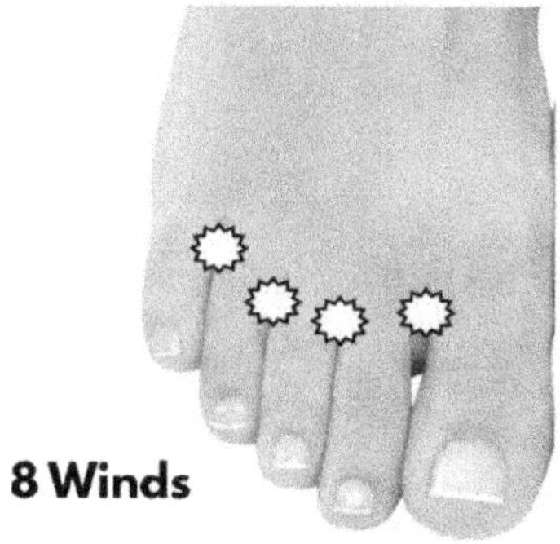

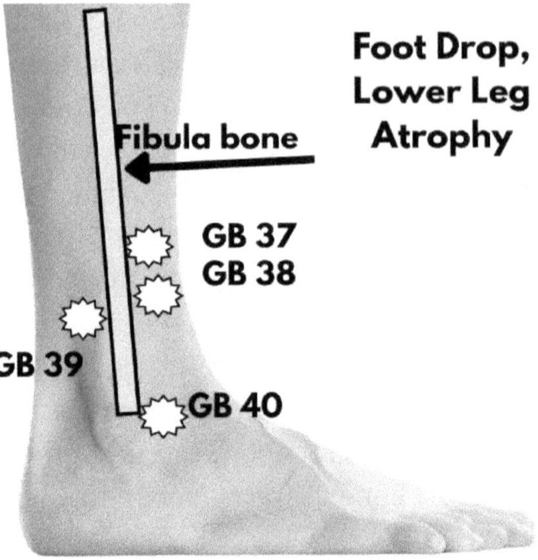

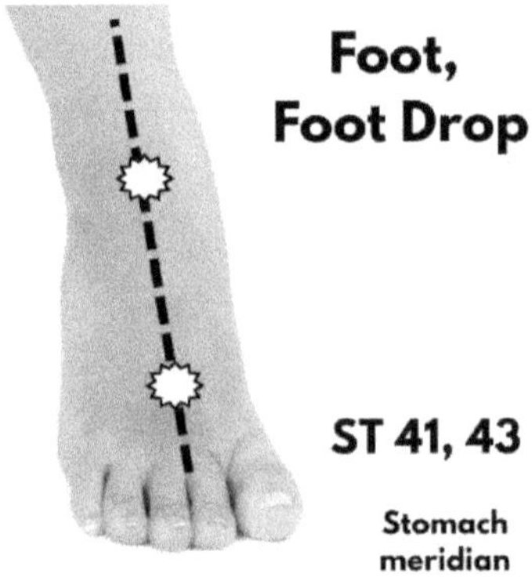

Stomach 41 is located at the ankle, at the level of the lateral malleolus, or outside ankle bone. It is in the hollow between the tendons. It treats foot drop, foot pain, lower leg pain, atrophy, and stiffness.

Stomach 43 is located between the second, and third-foot bones. It treats foot drop, foot pain or swelling, and toe pain or stiffness. To find this point, start at the area between the second and third toes, and glide your finger up your foot until you find a slight dip.

Spleen 6 is located 3 cun above the tip of the inner ankle bone, behind the tibia bone. Spleen 6 is one of the most important acupuncture points, because it has numerous functions. It treats edema, which is fluid retention. It treats hormonal imbalances, anxiety, and infertility. There are over 43 indications for this point in my point location book.

The most important function for this point to recover from a stroke is that it treats foot paralysis. It is a strong point, and you can sometimes feel the energy going down the inside of your foot when this point is stimulated. Press firmly just behind the tibia, or calf bone. Massage for about five minutes. There is no downside to massaging for longer. You will receive all the benefits of this point, in addition to helping to restore circulation in your lower leg and foot.

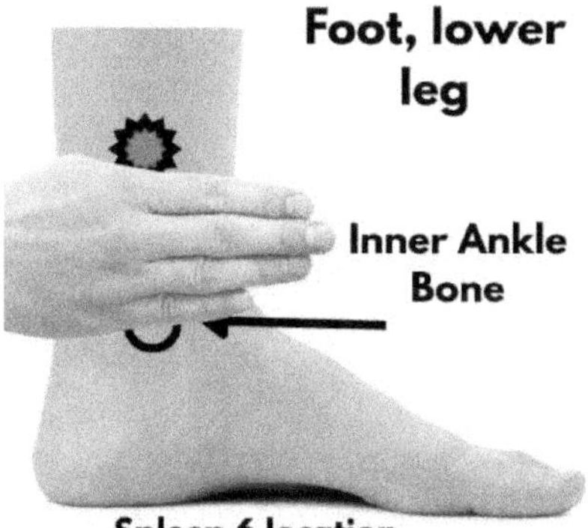

Spleen 6 location

Plantarflexion and dorsiflexion are caused by tight muscles in the lower legs. This can occur right after the stroke, or months or years later. When you have a problem with the movement of a limb, think about what muscles are affected. Heat up the muscles, and keep them warm. Do firm acupressure for 5-10 minutes while the muscles are warm.

For problems with the foot, always treat the gastrocnemius and soleus muscles, on the back of the calf. Regardless of the type of problem, these muscles need to be warmed and relaxed. Use a heating pad, hot water bottle, or electric blanket to warm the legs.

Gastrocnemius Muscle

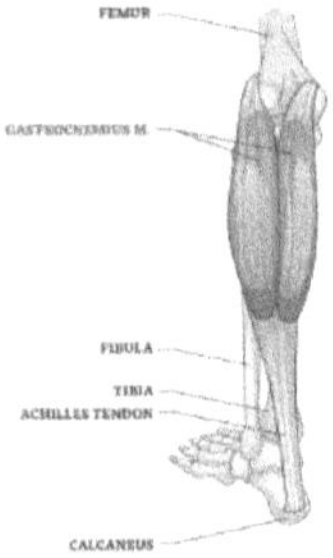

Soleus Muscle

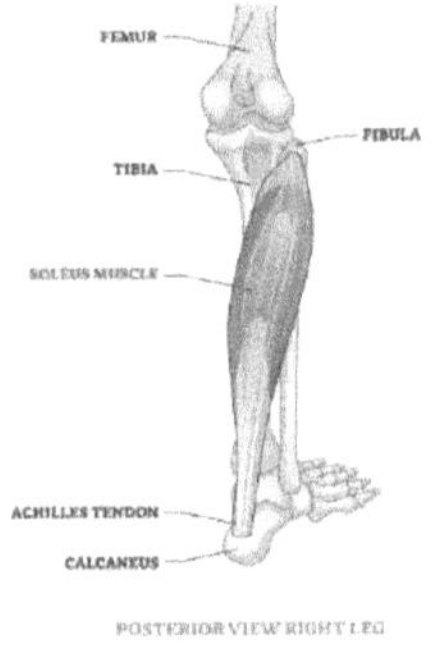

Cold Leg

Strokes can sometimes cause the limb to be cold. This happened to my dad. I used moxibustion on his calf muscles for over an hour. You MUST warm the muscles back up. If it is cold, circulation cannot be restored. Apply a heating pad, hot water bottle, or a ThermaCare patch to keep the muscles warm. I used the neck patch.

Even if your leg is not cold, keeping the legs warm will help to restore circulation to the area. When my mom was in the hospital, and I left for the day, I made sure she had ThermaCare patches on her arm, and lower legs. Anything you can do to stimulate an area would theoretically increase the brain's recognition of that area. So the acupressure, massage, acupuncture, or heat are all helpful. Heat also stimulates the area, so the brain notices it is there.

Do not worry about which points to use while you are warming up the affected area. Just keep it warm, and massage deeply into the muscles. Be careful not to overheat an area. You might not have full sensation in the area. The goal is not to super heat the muscles, but gently warm them and keep them warm to restore circulation.

Heating pads are designed to shut off after a certain number of hours. I also like hot water bottles. They stay hot longer and you can put them under your covers and keep the whole area warm. They are great to use locally on the affected area, or put under your covers at night to keep your feet and legs warm. You can find extra-large hot water bottles online, which cover a larger area. Electric throws stay warm for longer than electric blankets or heating pads.

Claw Toes

This section covers claw toes, or curled toes. The toes can curl up, or under the foot. Claw toes happen to to about 46% of patients who suffer a stroke.

There are several types of claw toe. It is also called toe flexion deformity, or digital flexor spasticity. The toes can curl up, or down.

After you have treated your legs and feet, as per the points in those sections, there are some additional points to try. These are not acupuncture points. I analyzed the muscles that lift the toes, and those that cause the toes to curl under, and you will find images of the legs and feet that show you where the best place is to treat. This is often where the muscles attach to the bone, or close to it. It depends on the surrounding anatomy.

Some people suffer from this temporarily, and some have lasting effects.

Three Main Types of Curled Toes

Claw toe is when the middle joints of the four smaller toes bend downward, causing the tips of the toes to curl upward.

Mallet toe is when the toes bend at the closest joint to the toenail, causing the tip of the toe to curl downward.

Hammer toe affects the second toe, which bends downward due to muscle weakness or paralysis. This is caused by paralysis or weakness of the foot muscles.

Curled toe disorder can cause foot cramps when at rest, or walking. Open sores or ulcers on the toes due to pressure from the shoe not fitting, and difficulty walking. If the problem persists, it could lead to pressure sores or ulcers on the toes.

Some sources say to use ice therapy. Ice therapy tightens the muscles. Cold tightens muscles. Muscles need to be warm to relax. Curled toes are caused by tight muscles, which are not getting enough circulation. Warm the muscles, and do acupressure on them to get them to relax more, and the stimulation will restore the brain connection.

There is no downside to treating the whole foot. Using warming therapy will also stimulate the nerves. Be careful with temperature, test with your fingers before you put your foot in. You can also treat both feet at the same time.

Warm the Feet and Legs

When treating tight, or painful muscles, it is very important to warm the muscles to help them relax. Here are a few ways to do that. I am repeating this on purpose.

- Use an electric heated foot bath, some of them have massagers
- Use a foot soak bucket
- Use any container that will hold warm water, and keep the temperature warm enough to relax the muscles
- Use a heating pad

After your feet and calves are thoroughly warm, you can either use your hands to massage, or use an acupressure mini massager, or any type of massager. The goal is to stimulate the nerves to restore the connection to your brain.

You can also add Epsom salts, or other types of herbal foot soaks, whatever feels comfortable to you.

Muscles That Lift Toes Upward

The main muscles that lift the toes upward (known as extension or dorsiflexion) are located in the front of the calf. These muscles include the **extensor digitorum longus**, **extensor hallucis longus**, and **extensor digitorum brevis**. If these muscles are shortened, or in spasm, the toes will go up.

The **tibialis anterior** muscle is called the foot drop muscle by the doctor who developed the theory on trigger points, Dr. Janet Travell.

Symptoms of a problem with this muscle are big toe pain, ankle hurts to move, dragging of the toes, or ankle weakness. Tripping or falling when walking can occur, due to the muscle not lifting the foot properly.

To make this simple, I have made images showing steps. Treating the tibialis anterior, shown in the image, will treat two other muscles that affect the foot, the extensor digitorum longus, and extensor hallucis longus. These muscles are right by your shin bone, which is the tibia bone, on the outside, or lateral part of leg. You need to press firmly enough to stimulate all the points.

Just start at the top, and move your way down. These are not acupuncture points, they are extra points to treat the muscle. They go along the stomach meridian in Chinese medicine. Most acupuncturists would automatically treat the Stomach meridian.

Step 1 is to treat the front of the calf, along the bone. You probably will not need step 2, but it is available to you in case you need it. You treat the muscles on the top of the foot, that is the extensor digitorum brevis.

Muscles That Curl Toes Downward

The muscle primarily responsible for curling your toes is the **flexor digitorum longus**. While several muscles in the leg and foot work together to control toe movement, the following are the most critical for curling:

Flexor Digitorum Longus: This deep muscle in the posterior leg (calf area) is the main driver for flexing (curling downward) the four **smaller toes**. **Flexor Hallucis Longus**: This muscle is specifically responsible for curling the **big toe**. It attaches to the fibula bone, which means you have to treat the outer part of the calf.

Flexor Digitorum Brevis: Located on the bottom of the foot, this muscle also assists in curling the four smaller toes. **Quadratus Plantae**: This muscle assists the flexor digitorum longus by correcting its pull and increasing its curling force. It is located on the bottom of the foot.

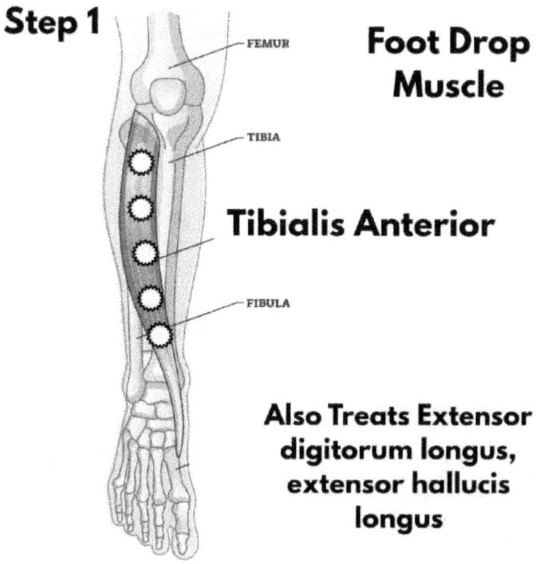

Step 2

Foot or Toe Drop

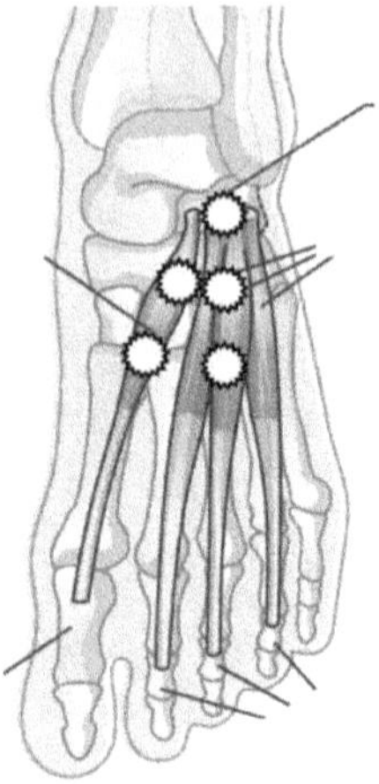

Extensor Digitorum Brevis

Top of Foot

Flexor Digitorum Longus Muscle

Step 1

Claw Toes

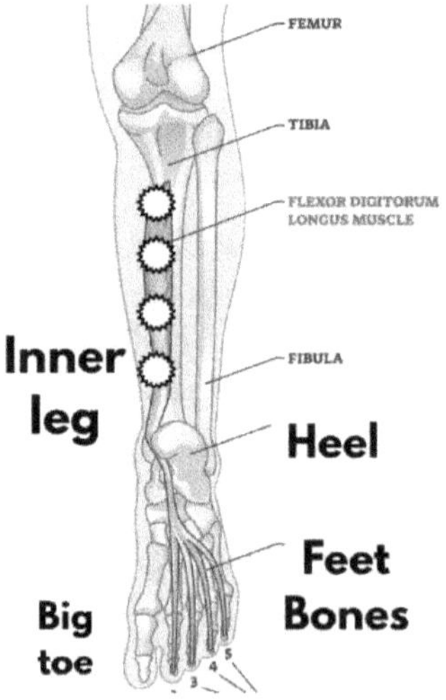

<u>Back of Calf</u>

Curls Toes Downward

Also treats flexor hallucis longus - big toe

Flexor Hallucis Longus

Claw Toes

Step 2

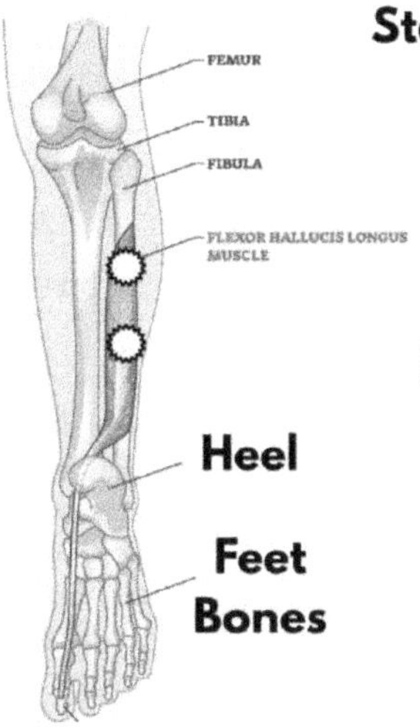

Big Toe

<u>Back of Calf</u>

Toe Curling, Claw Toe

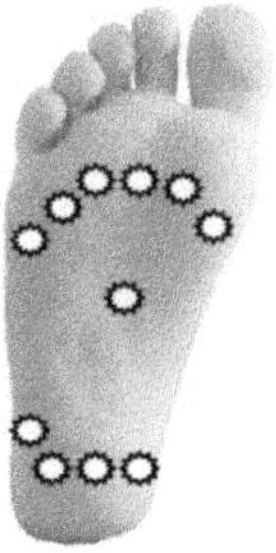

Toes Curled Under

Extra Points

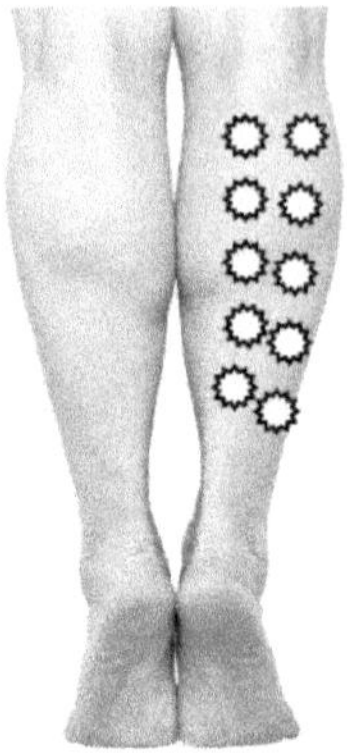

Claw toes

Treats flexor digitorum longus, flexor hallucis longus

CHAPTER 8

SPASTICITY AND CONTRACTURE

Stroke spasticity is a common, often painful complication which is described as involuntary muscle stiffness and spasms, affecting 30–80% of survivors. It is caused by brain signals failing to properly regulate the muscles.

This section is about general spasticity. Please refer to each section for specific areas. Spasticity can appear at any time after a stroke, but it is most common within 1-3 months after a stroke. That is one reason it is so important for you to treat your symptoms until they are completely resolved.

There is a chance that a new problem might occur a few years after your stroke. Just treat the points in this book, regardless of when spasticity occurs. Your brain is healing, and it tries to regulate function forever. That is why new symptoms could pop up several years later. That is also why you can continue to heal forever.

Spasticity, and muscle spasms, if not treated and resolved, can lead to contractures, where the muscle shortens and tightens up, which can reduce the ability to move the affected area.

Spasticity Symptoms

- Mild muscle stiffness
- Severe muscle stiffness, which can include frozen joints due to tight muscles
- When not used, the muscles shrink and shorten over time, which inhibits full range of motion
- Stiff fingers, arms, or legs
- Muscles spontaneously tighten up and relax, without your ability to control it
- Muscles fatigue easily, tight muscles restrict blood flow and oxygenation
- The joints can be deformed or frozen over time
- Clenched fist
- Tight fingers
- Arm can be bent and held against the chest
- Knee tightness
- Leg scissoring, which is involuntary crossing
- Foot that is bent at an angle
- A weakened foot that drags, making it hard to walk, also called foot drop
- Curled toes that make it hard to walk, also known as claw toe

In my research on what types of treatment patients get, I discovered that Botox injections are sometimes used. This paralyzes the muscles. Of course, it doesn't solve the underlying problem. After Botox is injected, acupuncture and other modalities will have little effect, because the nerves and muscles are basically frozen, and they will not respond to therapy. That is my experience. Once the Botox wears off, in about three months, regular therapy can be used, so don't despair.

Broken Bones and Frozen Muscles

Recently I broke my arm. After the bone had healed, the muscles around the broken area were frozen. They had frozen in place during the healing of the bone, but after the bone had healed, the muscles were still as hard as a rock. The thing that helped me the most was to apply heat eight hours a day. I believe the frozen muscles in my arm are similar to the frozen muscles stroke patients have.

I used a ThermaCare heat patch. I wrapped it around my arm, and left it on as long as it remained warm. It took about two months for the muscles to fully relax, but that alone was enough to release the muscles so I could move again.

If I did not use a ThermaCare heat wrap, I was not able to lift my arm to type, without a lot of pain. I wore a new ThermaCare patch every day, which enabled me to work. If you don't want to use ThermaCare heat patches, you can use a heating pad or heated throw on the affected area. Any time you can, apply gentle heat to the area. Keep applying it every chance you get, then try to stretch the spastic limb. Warm the muscle and stretch, as often as possible. Be gentle, do not force the muscles.

Keep Muscles Warm

Cold muscles cannot get adequate blood flow. Cold constricts blood flow. Do not allow your arms, legs, or other areas to stay cold. Keep everything warm.

Neither of my parents had spasticity. I believe it was because they both got acupuncture after their strokes, which restored circulation quickly.

To treat spasticity, and contracture, you should treat the spinal nerves. This is what I found in my research. These points are great for back pain, and are used all the time by acupuncturists, in addition to other points.

There are acupuncture points on either side of the spine, below the spinous process. Don't worry about getting the location right. Just heat and massage the areas on both sides of your spine. These points strongly stimulate the spinal nerves to improve circulation, and relax the muscles.

Before you do massage, make sure to warm the area for 15-30 minutes. If you massage cold muscles, it will not only not work as well, but you might be more prone to injure the tissue.

You can use any brand of massager, look for personal massager at your local store, or online. A larger head is better, because it can cover a larger area. If you use a wand massager, you can reach around and treat your own back.

I would not recommend a percussion massager. I think that is too rough. It could damage your muscles and nerves. You might not have full sensation right now, and you might not be aware when you are injuring yourself. You just need heat, and a gentle massager to restore blood flow.

You can also treat the spinal nerves in the upper back to make sure the upper back is not the cause of the problem. The problem can originate anywhere on the spine. Heat and massage are basically free. You can do it while you watch TV and you don't need help.

Spasticity

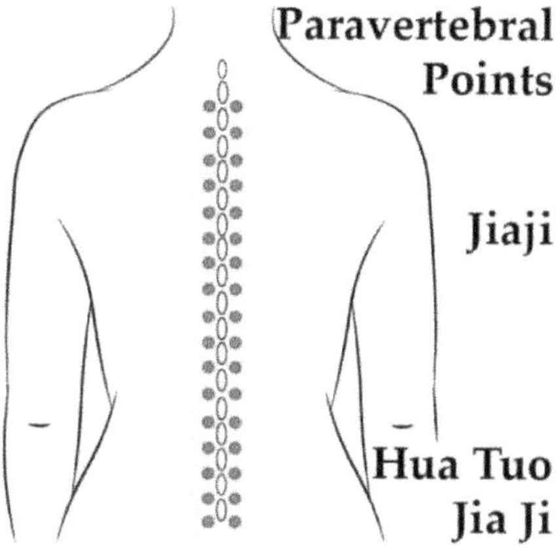

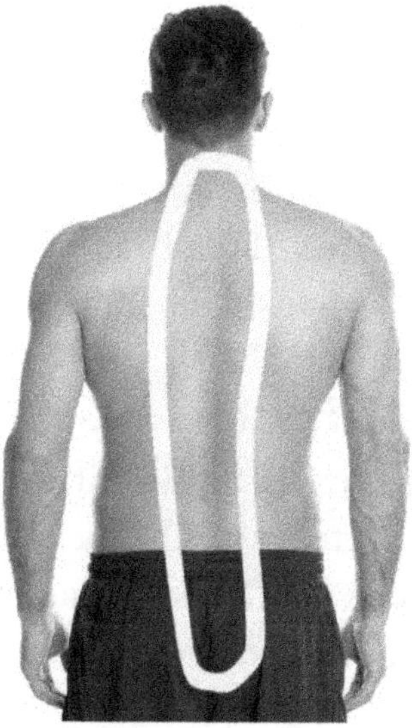

Spasticity

Warm and massage the entire spinal area

CHAPTER 9

STROKE PREVENTION

There are many possible causes of a stroke. The most common type of stroke, which is caused by a clot, causes about 88% of all strokes. So anything you can do to prevent a clot will reduce the odds of a stroke. The other type of stroke, which is hemorrhagic, is caused by a burst blood vessel in the brain. This is actually the easiest thing to prevent, using simple supplements. You can strengthen your blood vessels.

I will tell you the mainstream information on how to prevent a stroke, then I will tell you about additional things to consider, and supplements you can take to help yourself.

Key Risk Factors

- High blood pressure is the leading risk factor. It puts a strain on artery walls, which damages, and scars them, which can lead to plaque buildup. It can also weaken the blood vessels until they burst.
- Diabetes damages blood vessels, which increases stroke risk.
- High blood sugar levels make blood too thick
- Smoking damages blood vessels, and raises blood pressure

- Heart disease, which includes atrial fibrillation, which is an irregular heartbeat, can create clots that travel to the brain.
- High cholesterol is commonly cited by doctors as causing plaque that clogs arteries.
- Physical inactivity and obesity both increase overall stroke risk.
- Diet can increase stroke risk, especially high salt intake, and excess alcohol consumption, which can both raise blood pressure.

High Blood Pressure

High blood pressure damages the heart over time, and leads to heart arrhythmias, which can easily cause blood clots. A short term solution is to see your doctor for medication. Please do not ignore high blood pressure. Reduce stress as much as possible. Many people ignore high blood pressure, or don't even know they have it. This is the number one risk factor.

There is no magic bullet to control blood pressure. Treating stress and keeping it under control are the first step. Insulin resistance can cause high blood pressure. Keeping blood sugar stable is important.

Sleep Apnea

Sleep apnea has many possible causes. In Chinese medicine, snoring is caused by excess phlegm. Sleep apnea is a disease separate from snoring in modern medicine, but Chinese medicine would see the symptoms as similar. Eating foods that cause excess mucus production will cause snoring.

Dairy causes phlegm in Chinese medicine. All dairy. Most people do not have the enzymes necessary to digest dairy, so it causes an immune response, which causes excess mucus production in the sinuses and throat. It obstructs the airway by inflammation and mucus production.

If you stop eating all dairy, you should notice a difference in about a week. Food allergies or sensitivities like wheat or corn are also potentially involved with mucus production. Any time you increase allergies, you can increase mucus and swelling that can obstruct breathing. You will find you might sleep a lot better if you reduce or eliminate food allergens. Eggs and nuts are common allergens, look for congestion or sneezing after you eat.

Atrial Fibrillation

Atrial fibrillation is a common cause of stroke. It is a type of arrythmia. This would be seen in Chinese medicine as palpitations, which is often caused by weak heart energy. Herbal formulas such as Gui Pi Tang are given to make the heart stronger, so it can pump effectively. Your Licensed Acupuncturist can prescribe herbal formulas. Panax ginseng strengthens the heart, so if you have high blood pressure, avoid taking this. Codonopsis is a substitute for ginseng.

Other supplements to strengthen the heart include CoQ10, L-Carnitine, D-ribose, and magnesium. Hawthorn Berry extract has been improving heart function for centuries. It makes the heart stronger. It is a gentle heart tonic that can be taken by most people.

An excellent book on improving heart health is *Reverse Heart Disease Now*, by Dr. Stephen T. Sinatra. He recommends numerous supplements to prevent heart disease and stroke.

An estimated 8 million people in the US have atrial fibrillation, many do not know they have it. Up to 20% of strokes are related to atrial fibrillation. One in four adults over 40 years of age will develop atrial fibrillation in their lifetime.

Soft drinks contain phosphoric acid, which must be buffered by the minerals calcium, magnesium, and potassium. The acid drains your body of minerals. Your body pulls minerals from your blood and bones to buffer the acid. This can cause osteoporosis, and heart arrhythmias.

Atrial Fibrillation =
5x Stroke Risk

(Afib)

Weak Blood Vessels

It is hard to know if you have weak blood vessels. Easy bruising is a common symptom. When I treat patients with acupuncture, I can tell if someone has weak blood vessels, because they are more likely to bleed when the needles are removed. About 10% of my patients have weak blood vessels. I always tell them that the quality of your blood vessels in your legs is the same quality as the blood vessels in your brain and heart.

The best supplement to treat weak blood vessels is Diosmin. This is a bioflavanoid derived from citrus fruit. It strengthens the veins in a few days. I use Doctor's Best Vein Factors. You don't need the other ingredients some other supplement companies include in their vein products. It is also important to take vitamin C, and bioflavanoids.

Atherosclerosis

This is not commonly known, but one way to remove plaque in the arteries is to use Vitamin C, lysine, proline in equal amounts. Dr. Linus Pauling, who was a scientist with two Nobel prizes, discovered that coronary artery disease is caused by a vitamin C deficiency, which weakens artery walls, which causes Lipoprotein a, made by the body, to be sent to repair the blood vessels. Vitamin C and lysine are important to form collagen. They were able to show that supplemental vitamin C, lysine, and proline, were able to reverse atherosclerotic plaque.

The dosage recommended by Dr. Thomas E. Levy in his book, *Stop America's #1 Killer* is as follows:

Vitamin C: 3,000 to 9,000 mg daily, L-Lysine: 3,000 to 6,000 daily, and L-proline: 500 to 1,500 daily

Take this in divided doses. I have found many different doses online, but Dr. Levy is a vitamin C expert, who has written numerous books on using vitamin C medicinally, so I will quote him. His website is www.TomLevyMD.com.

You can buy your Lysine and Proline as individual supplements, or you can try Carlson Pro-Rite, which has equal amounts of lysine and proline. Combine that with equal amounts of vitamin C.

RESEARCH

The following research links should be considered as a reference only, for those interested in finding research on this topic. Most of the information in this book was derived from acupuncture textbooks. There is no right or wrong choice of acupuncture points.

There are many types of acupuncture. A few types are Traditional Chinese Medicine, Korean Medicine, Japanese Medicine, Tung acupuncture, Scalp acupuncture, Abdominal acupuncture, Ear acupuncture, and Hand acupuncture. There are many ways acupuncture can be used to treat health problems.

Meridian Names

If you do research on acupuncture, you will notice that acupuncture meridians can have different names. Most acupuncturists will use the Chinese Pin Yin name for the meridian. In China, the Chinese name for the point is used, the point numbering system is easier for non-Chinese speakers to remember.

The Du meridian is also called the Governing Vessel, abbreviated as GV. The Ren meridian is also called the Conception Vessel, abbreviated as CV. The San Jiao meridian is also called the Triple Warmer meridian, abbreviated as TW. There are also extra points which are not located on meridians, so they are called by their Chinese names, such as Yin Tang, Tai Yang, etc.

Aphasia

Li B, Deng S, Zhuo B, Sang B, Chen J, Zhang M, Tian G, Zhang L, Du Y, Zheng P, Yue G, Meng Z. Effect of Acupuncture vs Sham Acupuncture on Patients With Poststroke Motor Aphasia: A Randomized Clinical Trial. JAMA Netw Open. 2024 Jan 2;7(1):e2352580. doi: 10.1001/jamanetworkopen.2023.52580. PMID: 38252438; PMCID: PMC10804271.

Zhuo B, Deng S, Li B, Zhu W, Zhang M, Qin C, Meng Z. Possible Effects of Acupuncture in Poststroke Aphasia. Behav Neurol. 2023 Apr 12;2023:9445381. doi: 10.1155/2023/9445381. PMID: 37091130; PMCID: PMC10115536.

Li G, Yang ES. An fMRI study of acupuncture-induced brain activation of aphasia stroke patients. Complement Ther Med. 2011 Jan;19 Suppl 1:S49-59. doi: 10.1016/j.ctim.2010.11.004. Epub 2010 Dec 23. PMID: 21195295.

Li LL, Liu XW, Wu F, Tong DC, Ye LP, Tao HX, Liu P, Qiu YH, Yang WZ. Electroacupuncture Stimulation of Language-Implicated Acupoint Tongli (HT 5) in Healthy Subjects: An fMRI Evaluation Study. Chin J Integr Med. 2018 Nov;24(11):822-829. doi: 10.1007/s11655-017-2924-8. Epub 2017 Dec 11. PMID: 29230621.

Li B, Deng S, Sang B, Zhu W, Zhuo B, Zhang M, Qin C, Lyu Y, Du Y, Meng Z. Revealing the Neuroimaging Mechanism of Acupuncture for Poststroke Aphasia: A Systematic Review. Neural Plast. 2022 Apr 21;2022:5635596. doi: 10.1155/2022/5635596. PMID: 35494482; PMCID: PMC9050322.

Brain Recovery

Feng L, He W, Huang G, Lin S, Yuan C, Cheng H, He J, Liu Y. Reduced thiamine is a predictor for cognitive impairment of cerebral infarction. Brain Behav. 2020 Sep;10(9):e01709. doi: 10.1002/brb3.1709. Epub 2020 Aug 5. PMID: 32755028; PMCID: PMC7507112.

Wang WW, Xie CL, Lu L, Zheng GQ. A systematic review and meta-analysis of Baihui (GV20)-based scalp acupuncture in experimental ischemic stroke. Sci Rep. 2014 Feb 5;4:3981. doi: 10.1038/srep03981. PMID: 24496233; PMCID: PMC5379241.

Pan X, Gong N, Zhao J, Yu Z, Gu F, Chen J, Sun X, Zhao L, Yu M, Xu Z, Dong W, Qin Y, Fei G, Zhong C, Xu TL. Powerful beneficial effects of benfotiamine on cognitive impairment and beta-amyloid deposition in amyloid precursor protein/presenilin-1 transgenic mice. Brain. 2010 May;133(Pt 5):1342-51. doi: 10.1093/brain/awq069. Epub 2010 Apr 12. PMID: 20385653.

Zhang Y, Tang YW, Peng YT, Yan Z, Zhou J, Yue ZH. Acupuncture, an effective treatment for post-stroke neurologic dysfunction. Brain Res Bull. 2024 Sep;215:111035. doi: 10.1016/j.brainresbull.2024.111035. Epub 2024 Jul 26. PMID: 39069104.

Li K, Shi G, Zhao Y, Chen Y, Gao J, Yao L, Zhao J, Li H, Xu Y, Chen Y. Electroacupuncture Ameliorates Neuroinflammation-Mediated Cognitive Deficits through Inhibition of NLRP3 in Presenilin1/2 Conditional Double Knockout Mice. Neural Plast. 2021 Jan 6;2021:8814616. doi: 10.1155/2021/8814616. PMID: 33505459; PMCID: PMC7806385.

Chen J, Wang J, Huang Y, Lai X, Tang C, Yang J, Wu J, Zeng T, Qu S. Modulatory effect of acupuncture at Waiguan (TE5) on the functional connectivity of the central nervous system of patients with ischemic stroke in the left basal ganglia. PLoS One. 2014 Jun 13;9(6):e96777. doi: 10.1371/journal.pone.0096777. PMID: 24927275; PMCID: PMC4057077.

Chen J, Huang Y, Lai X, Tang C, Yang J, Chen H, Zeng T, Wu J, Qu S. Acupuncture at Waiguan (TE5) influences activation/deactivation of functional brain areas in ischemic stroke patients and healthy people: A functional MRI study. Neural Regen Res. 2013 Jan 25;8(3):226-32. doi: 10.3969/j.issn.1673-5374.2013.03.004. PMID: 25206592; PMCID: PMC4107521.

Shi P, Sun LL, Lee YS, Tu Y. Electroacupuncture regulates the stress-injury-repair chain of events after cerebral ischemia/reperfusion injury. Neural Regen Res. 2017 Jun;12(6):925-930. doi: 10.4103/1673-5374.208574. PMID: 28761425; PMCID: PMC5514867.

Bladder Infections – Olive Leaf Extract

Esfandiary MA, Khosravi AR, Asadi S, Nikaein D, Hassan J, Sharifzadeh A. Antimicrobial and anti-biofilm properties of oleuropein against Escherichia coli and fluconazole-resistant isolates of Candida albicans and Candida glabrata. BMC Microbiol. 2024 May 4;24(1):154. doi: 10.1186/s12866-024-03305-5. PMID: 38704559; PMCID: PMC11069153.

B Vitamins and Choline

Folic acid impacts neuroplasticity. After ischemic damage, stroke, the mice that received B vitamins and choline had increased levels of BDNF, compared to control mice. BDNF is brain derived neurotrophic factor, which is a factor showing brain cell growth. Folic acid reduces the risk of stroke in adults. Animals deficient in vitamin B 12 have reduced levels of neurotrophic factors.

Jadavji NM, Emmerson JT, MacFarlane AJ, Willmore WG, Smith PD. B-vitamin and choline supplementation increases neuroplasticity and recovery after stroke. Neurobiol Dis. 2017 Jul;103:89-100. doi: 10.1016/j.nbd.2017.04.001. Epub 2017 Apr 7. PMID: 28396257.

B 12 Vitamin

Vitamin B 12 deficiency increases homocysteine in the blood, which increases the chance for a stroke. B 12 deficiency worsens stroke outcome. Up to 40% of people are deficient in vitamin B 12. B 12 is usually derived from animal protein in the diet, but as we age, our digestion declines, which means we cannot extract the nutrients we need for healthy function.

B 12 is also specific to nervous tissue.

Vitamin B 12 supplements can be hard to absorb and the dosage is too low to make a difference. I have seen fast results by taking 5,000 mcg dosage liquid. Two droppers three times daily will quickly address deficiencies. Some people want to take B 12 shots. shots. If you can get your doctor to do that for you, that's great. But with the easy availability of high dose B 12 supplements, I can't see a reason to do that.

Taking B 12 liquid orally means that you just drop it in your mouth, and it is absorbed through the tissue in your mouth. Make sure to take Methylcobalamin, not Cyanocobalamin. Methylcobalamin is better absorbed and there are no known side effects.

Vitamin B 12 deficiency can be a risk factor in dementia and Alzheimer's. B 12 reduces homocysteine, which reduces stroke risk.

Mbs GBY, Wasek B, Bottiglieri T, Malysheva O, Caudill MA, Jadavji NM. Dietary vitamin B12 deficiency impairs motor function and changes neuronal survival and choline metabolism after ischemic stroke in middle-aged male and female mice. Nutr Neurosci. 2024 Apr;27(4):300-309. doi: 10.1080/1028415X.2023.2188639. Epub 2023 Mar 17. PMID: 36932327.

"One study showed that B 12 therapy slowed gray matter atrophy and cognitive decline in the Homocysteine and B vitamins Cognitive Impairment Trial. Undiagnosed metabolic B 12 deficiency may be an important missed opportunity for prevention of dementia and stroke."

Spence JD. Metabolic vitamin B12 deficiency: a missed opportunity to prevent dementia and stroke. Nutr Res. 2016 Feb;36(2):109-16. doi: 10.1016/j.nutres.2015.10.003. Epub 2015 Oct 21. PMID: 26597770.

One study said that Vitamin B 12 deficiency leads to the accumulation of atherogenic homocysteine, a well-known risk factor for ischemic stroke. Vitamin B 12, combined with B vitamins, dramatically reduced stroke, myocardial infarction, and vascular death by 34% in patients without renal impairment.

Vitamin B 12 deficient mice exhibited larger infarct sizes. (Infarct is the area of damage in the brain).

Mice given vitamin B 12 showed a better survival rate and a significantly smaller infarct volume compared to Vitamin B 12 deficient mice. It also significantly alleviated stroke induced neurological impairment. The mice given vitamin B 12 showed much better recovery of sensorimotor function after stroke.

Vitamin B 12 globally reduced neuroinflammation.

Ge Y, Yang C, Zadeh M, Sprague SM, Lin YD, Jain HS, Determann BF 2nd, Roth WH, Palavicini JP, Larochelle J, Candelario-Jalil E, Mohamadzadeh M. Functional regulation of microglia by vitamin B12 alleviates ischemic stroke-induced neuroinflammation in mice. iScience. 2024 Mar 14;27(4):109480. doi: 10.1016/j.isci.2024.109480. PMID: 38715940; PMCID: PMC11075062.

B3 Niacin

Niacin promotes synaptic plasticity and axon growth in the ischemic brain.

Cui X, Chopp M, Zacharek A, Roberts C, Buller B, Ion M, Chen J. Niacin treatment of stroke increases synaptic plasticity and axon growth in rats. Stroke. 2010 Sep;41(9):2044-9. doi: 10.1161/STROKEAHA.110.589333. Epub 2010 Jul 29. PMID: 20671245; PMCID: PMC2932778.

Constipation

Wang DS, Wang S, Kong LL, Wang WY, Cui XM. [Clinical observation on abdominal electroacupuncture for treatment of poststroke constipation]. Zhongguo Zhen Jiu. 2008 Jan;28(1):7-9. Chinese. PMID: 18257178.

Curcumin

Curcumin treatment significantly reduced infarct volume and improved neurological scores. Curcumin is used as a Chinese herb to treat blood stasis, which is thick blood. There are stronger herbs available, but curcumin is easy to find and less likely to cause side effects. The brand you use can make a big difference, I personally like Nature's Way, and Planetary Herbals.

Zhao J, Yu S, Zheng W, Feng G, Luo G, Wang L, Zhao Y. Curcumin improves outcomes and attenuates focal cerebral ischemic injury via antiapoptotic mechanisms in rats. Neurochem Res. 2010 Mar;35(3):374-9. doi: 10.1007/s11064-009-0065-y. Epub 2009 Sep 23. PMID: 19774461.

Curcumin significantly improved sensorimotor function, and reduced white matter lesion in the brain.

Ran Y, Su W, Gao F, Ding Z, Yang S, Ye L, Chen X, Tian G, Xi J, Liu Z. Curcumin Ameliorates White Matter Injury after Ischemic Stroke by Inhibiting Microglia/Macrophage Pyroptosis through NF-κB Suppression and NLRP3 Inflammasome Inhibition. Oxid Med Cell Longev. 2021 Sep 30;2021:1552127. doi: 10.1155/2021/1552127. PMID: 34630845; PMCID: PMC8497115.

Foot Drop

Jo HJ, Chae GE, Kim HW, Lee YJ, Koh A, Choi JE, Kim SJ, Kim WY. Electroacupuncture Treatment for Post-Stroke Foot Drop: A Systemic Review of Randomized Controlled Trials. J Acupunct Res 2024;41:75-86. https://doi.org/10.13045/jar.24.0002

Garlic – Stroke Prevention

Garlic lowers blood pressure by 7%, reduces blood clotting and stickiness. In a four-year trial, arteriosclerotic plaque volume reduced by 9-18%, with a 3% regression in plaque volume. These effects of garlic result in a reduction of relative cardiovascular risk for infarction and stroke by more than 50%. Note: I use Kyolic Reserve, which is pure, aged garlic.

Hiccups

Chang CC, Chang ST, Li TY, Chiang SL, Tsai KC, Lin JC. Resolution of intractable hiccups after near-infrared irradiation of relevant acupoints. Am J Med Sci. 2006 Aug;332(2):93-96. doi: 10.1097/00000441-200608000-00009. PMID: 16909058.

Incontinence

Cheng P, Chi Z, Xiao Y, Xie W, Zhu D, Yu T, Li H, Qin S, Jiao L. The acupuncture-related therapy for post-stroke urinary incontinence: A protocol for systematic review and network meta-analysis. Medicine (Baltimore). 2020 Oct 30;99(44):e22865. doi: 10.1097/MD.0000000000022865. PMID: 33126332; PMCID: PMC7598822.

Nattokinase

In one study, Nattokinase significantly reduced infarct volumes by 54-68%. This enzyme is commonly used to reduce and dissolve blood clots and relieve inflammation and pain. By dissolving blood clots, the tissue damage in the brain can be reduced.

One study demonstrates that NK protects against acute ischemic stroke and impressively promotes neurogenesis in rat models by increasing peripheral blood irisin, leading to improved cognitive function.

Wu H, Zhang Q, Xu P, Chen J, Duan L, Xu F, Zhang F. Nattokinase Promotes Post-stroke Neurogenesis and Cognition Recovery via Increasing Circulating Irisin. J Agric Food Chem. 2023 Aug 2;71(30):11418-11428. doi: 10.1021/acs.jafc.2c08718. Epub 2023 Jul 19. PMID: 37466380.

Nattokinase can break down blood clots by directly hydrolyzing fibrin and plasmin substrate. Unlike common fibrinolytic proteases, pharmaceuticals, which can produce various side effects such as bleeding, nattokinase exhibits little to no side effects.

A 26 week study compared Nattokinase enzyme, with a statin drug. The reduction in plaque size in the nattokinase group was 36.6%. In the statin group, the plaque reduction was only 11.5%.

Ren NN, Chen HJ, Li Y, Mcgowan GW, Lin YG. [A clinical study on the effect of nattokinase on carotid artery atherosclerosis and hyperlipidaemia]. Zhonghua Yi Xue Za Zhi. 2017 Jul 11;97(26):2038-2042. Chinese. doi: 10.3760/cma.j.issn.0376-2491.2017.26.005. PMID: 28763875.

Wang, J.-M & Chen, H.-Y & Cheng, S.-M & Chen, S.-H & Yang, L.-L & Cheng, F.-C. (2012). Nattokinase Reduces Brain Infarction, Fibrinogen and Activated Partial Thromboplastin Time against Cerebral Ischemia-Reperfusion Injury. Journal of Food and Drug Analysis. 20. 686-691+717. 10.6227/jfda.2012200317.

Spasticity

Li H, Long D, Li B, Liu H, Ma T, Wu T, Eriksson M, Wen Y, Wei J, You W, Liu Y, Xu X, Zhang Y, Wang L, Sun J. A clinical study to assess the influence of acupuncture at "Wang's Jiaji" acupoints on limb spasticity in patients in convalescent stage of ischemic stroke: study protocol for a randomized controlled trial. Trials. 2019 Jul 10;20(1):419. doi: 10.1186/s13063-019-3464-7. PMID: 31291976; PMCID: PMC6621988.

Shi P, Sun LL, Lee YS, Tu Y. Electroacupuncture regulates the stress-injury-repair chain of events after cerebral ischemia/reperfusion injury. Neural Regen Res. 2017 Jun;12(6):925-930. doi: 10.4103/1673-5374.208574. PMID: 28761425; PMCID: PMC5514867.

Swallowing – Dysphagia

Qin L, Zhang XP, Yang XC, Cui CH, Shi J, Jia CS. [Deep acupuncture of Lianquan (CV23) and Yifeng (TE17) in combination with conventional acupuncture of other acupoints is superior to swallowing rehabilitation training in improving post-stroke dysphagia in apoplexy patients]. Zhen Ci Yan Jiu. 2019 Feb

25;44(2):144-7. Chinese. doi: 10.13702/j.1000-0607.180018. PMID: 30945493.

The following report indicates that combining traditional swallowing training, and acupuncture led to an effective rate of 94.92%.

Cui S, Yao S, Wu C, Yao L, Huang P, Chen Y, Tang C, Xu N. Electroacupuncture Involved in Motor Cortex and Hypoglossal Neural Control to Improve Voluntary Swallowing of Poststroke Dysphagia Mice. Neural Plast. 2020 Sep 27;2020:8857543. doi: 10.1155/2020/8857543. PMID: 33061953; PMCID: PMC7537716.

REFERENCES

Acupuncture Points Handbook, Deborah Bleecker

A Manual of Acupuncture by Peter Deadman (Author), Mazin Al-Khafaji (Author), Kevin Baker (Author)

Evidence -based Clinical Chinese Medicine, Volume 12, Post-Stroke Shoulder Complications, Claire Shuiqing Zhang, Shaonan Liu

Evidence-based Clinical Chinese Medicine, Volume 13, Post-Stroke Spasticity, Claire Shuiqing Zhang, Shaonan Liu

Acupuncture and Moxibustion for Stroke Rehabilitation by Fan Gang-Qi (Author), Wang Qi-cai (Author), Chen Ji (Translator), Ni Guang-Xia (Contributor)

Pubmed which is the US government website which compiles research from all over the world.
https://pubmed.ncbi.nlm.nih.gov/

INDEX

About the Author

Deborah Bleecker is a Licensed Acupuncturist, and has a Master of Science degree in Oriental Medicine, since 1999. She suffered a repetitive stress injury in 1994, and lived with chronic pain until she decided she would have to find her own answers to her health problems. Medical doctors told her that her pain was incurable, but she was able to recover with the help of acupuncture and Chinese medicine. She has written numerous books on health issues, including *Acupuncture Points Handbook*, and *Acupressure Made Simple.*

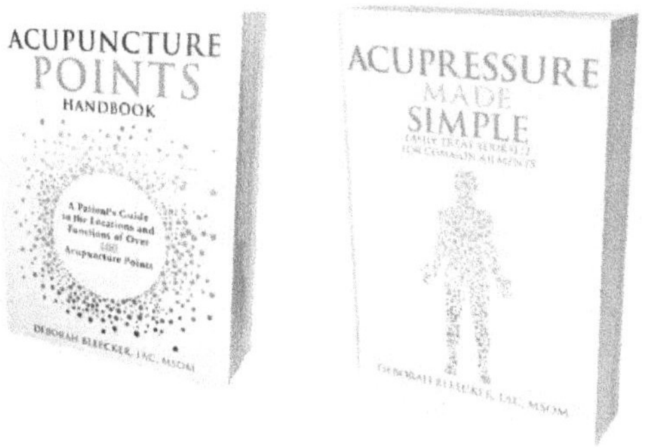

www.ingramcontent.com/pod-product-compliance
Lightning Source LLC
LaVergne TN
LVHW050819061126
851857LV00012B/885